Praise for Coping with Psoriasis

Being diagnosed with psoriasis can feel overwhelming. Coping with Psoriasis *explores the complexities of living with psoriasis, the everyday things that really matter to people, and offers sensible advice and solutions. Living with psoriasis can feel lonely, and in the book Dr Catherine O'Leary gently reassures the reader that their feelings towards psoriasis are both valid and understandable, offering her support and wisdom as a clinical psychologist and someone living with the condition. A must read for anyone affected by psoriasis.*

Helen McAteer, Chief Executive, Psoriasis Association

This is a really insightful and well-written book about the many psychological facets of living with a serious skin disease, namely psoriasis. It has been written by a consultant clinical psychologist, who not only has a lifetime of experience of living with psoriasis but is also able to draw upon an extensive body of research which has investigated the psychological impact of long-term physical health problems. This combination of personal, professional and scientific insights is the book's unique strength. What is so impressive is that Catherine shares many of her very personal experiences in an honest and open way, and then is able to make use of evidence-based psychological research and theory to explain why and how people's feelings, thoughts and social experiences can have such a profound effect on the impact of an illness such as psoriasis. Just as important as providing explanations of these psychological effects is all the practical advice for facilitating coping, which is succinctly summarised at the end of each chapter. This is a moving, powerful and useful book, which should be read by clinicians, patients and anyone wanting to understand more about the psychology of health and illness.

Professor John Weinman, Professor of Psychology as applied to Medicines, School of Cancer & Pharmaceutical Sciences, King's College London

Working as a Nurse Consultant specialising in psoriasis, this is a book I will be recommending for my patients. Many of my patients require support and have experienced a negative quality of life impacted by the burden of psoriasis. Catherine beautifully describes her journey with psoriasis since childhood, which will give hope to many as they will feel they are not alone. This is such a valuable book to read as both a healthcare professional and as a patient. There are fantastic strategies and top tips to help people cope with aspects of anxiety, stress and depression. Catherine writes about all aspects of living with psoriasis which include pain, self-loathing, relationships, cultural differences, stigma and top tips on coping with all. Another important chapter is advice for healthcare professionals to help them communicate with patients and acknowledge the psychological aspect of psoriasis. There are so many resources included in this book to help clinicians provide excellent care for patients with psoriasis, and I will be recommending my colleagues to read this book. I personally loved this book.

Teena Mackenzie, Consultant Nurse in Inflammatory Disease and Biologics, and Education and Development Lead for the British Dermatological Nursing Group

Unfortunately, people with psoriasis often don't have access to the same support available to people with other long-term conditions. As such, this book is much needed. Written by a Consultant Clinical Psychologist, Dr Catherine O'Leary, the book provides an up-to-date account of the complex relationship between psoriasis and psychological functioning. Dr O'Leary not only draws on her knowledge of the latest research but also movingly shares her personal experience of living with this highly visible and often painful condition. In doing so, she presents a compelling account of the relationship between the mind and the skin, and also the important role played by other people. Each chapter ends with straightforward and evidence-based self-help guidance and 'tips' (including importantly tips on managing other people). If you are living with psoriasis or interested in learning more about this condition, then I highly recommend this book as a source of support, wisdom and hopefulness.

Professor Andrew R Thompson, Consultant Clinical Psychologist and Psychodermatology Researcher

Coping with Psoriasis *is an engaging read that is a must for anyone whose life is impacted with psoriasis. Dr O'Leary provides a unique insight into the emotional and psychological effects of psoriasis with her personal experience and in her capacity as an experienced clinical psychologist.*

Lucy Moorhead, Nurse Consultant in Inflammatory Skin Disease, Guy's and St Thomas' NHS Foundation Trust

Psoriasis can be a life-ruining disease that even in the 21st century is immensely stigmatising for sufferers who often are unable to lead a normal life. Dr O'Leary has highlighted and crystallised the anguish and life course impairment of people with psoriasis but at the same time has produced practical tips to enable patients to cope with the disease. A very worthwhile read for patients as well as their family members and healthcare providers.

Professor Chris Griffiths OBE, Emeritus Professor of Dermatology, The University of Manchester

It was an honour to be asked to review this book, which I would thoroughly recommend to people living with psoriasis as well as their healthcare practitioners. There's something unique about hearing the perspective of someone who is a patient as well as a clinical expert in that field. Catherine's lived experiences of living with psoriasis shines through each chapter, full of top tips for helping others to manage their condition. Catherine's letter to herself as a 16-year-old at the end of the book is particularly poignant, full of insights, hope and wisdom.

Professor Delyth Higman James, Professor of Health Psychology in Pharmacy Practice and Principal Lead for REF (Health Sciences), Cardiff Metropolitan University

Coping with Psoriasis

Coping with Psoriasis

Understanding and navigating the emotional challenges

Dr Catherine O'Leary
Illustrations by Arianne Barratt

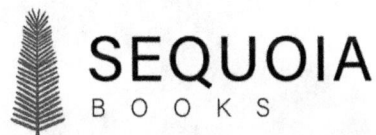

Every possible effort has been made to ensure that the information contained in this book is accurate at the time of going to press. The publishers and author(s) cannot accept responsibility for any errors and omissions, however caused. No responsibility for loss or damage occasioned to any person acting, or refraining from action, as a result of the material contained in this publication can be accepted by the editor, the publisher or the author.

First published in 2024 by Sequoia Books

Apart from fair dealing for the purposes of research or private study, or criticism or review, as permitted under the Copyright, Designs and Patents act 1988, this publication may only be reproduced, stored or transmitted, in any form or by any means, with the prior permission in writing of the publisher, or in the case of reprographic reproduction in accordance with the terms and licenses issued by the CLA. Enquiries concerning reproduction outside these terms should be sent to the publisher using the details on the website www.sequoia-books.com

©Catherine O'Leary 2024

The right of Catherine O'Leary to be identified as author of this work has been asserted in accordance with the Copyright, Designs and Patents act 1988.

ISBN
Print: 9781914110368
EPUB: 9781914110375

A CIP record for this book is available from the British Library

Library of Congress Cataloguing-In-Publication Data

Name: Catherine O'Leary
Title: Coping With Psoriasis
Description: 1st Edition, Sequoia Books UK 2024
Print: 9781914110368
EPUB: 9781914110375

Library of Congress Control Number: 2024911688

Print and Electronic production managed by Deanta Global

Contents

Figures xi
Foreword xii
The unique perspective xiii
Acknowledgements xv

1 Introduction   1
2 Psoriasis and depression   13
3 Psoriasis and stress   25
4 Psoriasis and shame   39
5 Dealing with unwanted attention and others' reactions   52
6 Living with pain, discomfort and itching   63
7 Blame and lifestyle factors   77
8 Psoriasis and emotions   88
9 Relationships and intimacy   100
10 Models of illness beliefs   113
11 Psychological strategies for coping   125
12 Developing self-compassion   140
13 Coping with treatments   153

14 Supporting others with psoriasis	165
15 Positive growth and psoriasis	179

Appendices

Resources	187
Mental health concerns	193
Letter to my younger self	197
References	199
Glossary of terms	210
About the author	213

Figures

1.1	Psoriasis iceberg	11
2.1	Symptoms of depression	15
2.2	Negative spiral of depression in psoriasis	21
3.1	Proposed pathway between stress and psoriasis	28
3.2	Vicious cycle of panic	32
4.1	The psoriasis compass of shame	45
5.1	The psoriasis Explain, Reassure, Distract technique	56
6.1	The psoriasis anger firework	66
6.2	Methods to close the gate and reduce the psoriasis pain signals	70
6.3	The complex relationship between psoriasis, pain and suffering	75
7.1	Potential factors triggering a flare-up	80
7.2	Challenges of following a virtuous cycle	85
8.1	Traits associated with alexithymia	91
8.2	Polyvagal theory	95
9.1	Different types of social support	106
10.1	Three-step problem-solving model	115
10.2	Case studies illustrating how illness beliefs can drive behaviour and feelings	120
11.1	Types of thinking errors	128
11.2	The defeated bus driver	133
11.3	The despairing bus driver	133
11.4	The ACT bus driver	134
12.1	How psoriasis can impact the emotional regulation system	145
13.1	Cycle of behaviour change	162

Foreword

Dr Sarah Swan
Coping with… Series Editor
Consultant Clinical Psychologist

When I was diagnosed with breast cancer in 2019, I knew I was going to have to use my skills as a clinical psychologist to help me cope with the distress that this inevitably caused. Early on in my journey, I had the urge to write, as a way of processing my experiences. I immediately thought it had the potential for a book, but never thought this would come to fruition. But with the support of the Association of Clinical Psychologists, Sequoia Publishing, friends, family and colleagues, I committed to writing the book.

I began to realise what a unique position I held: facing a difficult life event that many others face, but with the knowledge and experience of a long career in helping people with their emotional experiences. Suddenly, it dawned on me that there could be any number of difficult or challenging experiences that other clinical psychologists may have faced. And, like me, they would, in all likelihood, have valuable skills to share with others facing the same situation. And so, the idea for the series was born.

It is an honour to launch the series with my book, *Coping with Breast Cancer*. And it has been my pleasure to support other clinical psychologists with their writing in order to produce a series of books that will help to bring valuable psychological ideas to a wide audience. With the knowledge and skills of the writers, I am confident that this series will benefit many people facing difficult and challenging situations and give them helpful skills to cope.

The unique perspective

Dr Penelope Cream
Clinical and Health Psychologist
Director of Operations, ACP-UK

The Association of Clinical Psychologists UK (ACP-UK) is delighted to be publishing these important *Coping With…* books. In these pages, clinical psychologists have taken the courageous step of sharing how they applied their skills to their own lives, in order to help others facing similar difficulties and challenges.

The profession of clinical psychology spans many types of psychological approaches across all areas of the lifespan and of individual experiences, from physical health, psychological distress and mental illness, as well as cognitive difficulties, family challenges and workplace problems. Clinical psychologists have rigorous training not only in psychological therapies but also in research methods and using evidence-based practice. They draw on these aspects to inform everything they do, including looking after themselves. These books evidence the flexibility and creativity with which we can use and apply our skills, both to help ourselves and others.

It is not often that clinicians share their first-hand experiences of challenging situations and how they have applied what they have learnt in their training and the many years of experience that follow. I feel very proud of my clinical psychology colleagues who have written this series of books, not only for everything that they have experienced

The unique perspective

with courage and insight, but for the generosity and openness with which they want to help other people. It is not easy to combine subjective personal experience with an external clinical perspective, yet in these books, they share the breadth of knowledge and training that the profession brings us.

Acknowledgements

I've been lucky enough to have great family and friends around me as I've navigated life as a psychologist and someone with psoriasis, and I owe a huge debt of gratitude to every one of them. There are a few people who deserve special mention, including my colleagues and friends, Anna and Viv, who encouraged me to send a proposal for this book and were cheerleaders throughout the process. As someone who has perfected the art of hiding their skin, I don't think I would have had the courage to start writing without their support.

Thank you to my greatest joy, my children Dylan, Tudor and Arianne, who have never been the least bit bothered by my skin. Without their IT skills and artistic endeavours, my *Coping with Psoriasis* website and this book would have remained only a small seed of possibility. Special thanks to Arianne for turning my ideas and scribbles into the lovely illustrations you see in this book.

Finally, thanks to Jim for being by my side throughout my adult life. Thank you for listening to my ideas, reading all my drafts and believing in me no matter how flaky I feel.

1 Introduction

I'm so glad you've picked up this book. If, like me, you've had psoriasis for a long time, or if you've been recently diagnosed, you'll know that living with the condition is not at all easy. Besides dealing with the physical symptoms, psoriasis can have a significant psychological impact and present many challenges to your day-to-day life. I've written this book for people with psoriasis, for people living with those with psoriasis and for those who work with people with psoriasis. My aim is that it can be used alongside your treatments to help you cope with the condition and live a full and as happy a life as possible. My purpose in writing it is to not only provide insight and understanding about the psychological impact of psoriasis but also to suggest things that people with the condition can do to feel better about themselves.

I feel I'm in a unique position to write this book. Besides being a clinical psychologist, I also have psoriasis. This gives me both a clinical and a personal experience of what it's like to live with psoriasis.

I have both guttate and plaque psoriasis. The guttate patches are small and numerous, looking almost like someone has flicked a paintbrush dipped in red paint at my body. The plaque psoriasis is formed of larger patches covered with scaly skin. Right now, I have psoriasis on most of my scalp, in my ears and a small plaque on one side of my face. Both my arms, my back and my stomach are affected. I have a couple of new patches on my left wrist. I see them every time I look at my watch. Large plaques on my bottom are embarrassing and can make sitting down for long periods painful. Both my legs are affected, and I have a few patches on the soles of my feet. Most of the plaques on my body are small, around the size of a penny, but some are much larger. They are not overly red currently, which is a sign to me that it's not at its most active phase. When my skin is flaring, the plaques are deep, angry red and hot to the touch. The psoriatic patch is rough and raised, with thickened, peeling skin. When I take off my clothes, a snowstorm of skin flakes swirls around me. When I get up from a chair, I leave a dusting of skin behind. My scalp itches, as do the insides of my ears and one small but unreachable plaque between my shoulder blades. My toenails are pitted and thickened. My fingernails are pretty clear at the moment, except for my thumbnails which are grooved and with psoriasis down the sides, beneath the nail. The joints in my fingers and wrists hurt sporadically but right now they feel fine. I'm having a new pain in my lower back which I'm worrying might be a form of psoriatic arthritis (PsA).

If I'd have written this six months ago, the story would have been different. My skin was pretty clear then, and the plaques I did have were much paler. Six months before that and things were as bad as they get. The constantly changing severity of my skin means I routinely question what I'm doing differently, why it's changing and whether it's my fault. Did I eat the wrong thing, get too stressed, sleep too little, sleep too much? I worry how bad it's going to get in a week, a month and in six months.

Things only improve for me with a treatment like phototherapy or a holiday in the sun. As soon as I'm away from those healing UVB rays, it starts to get worse again. It's always getting worse but sometimes slowly, like right now, and other times it rages throughout my body and spreads at an alarming rate. I don't think there's a patch of my skin that hasn't had psoriasis at one time or another. I'm waiting for a space to start phototherapy in my local dermatology service and I'm hopeful this will control things for a while.

Psoriasis and me

My psoriasis began during childhood. I was born in the 1970s in South Wales, the middle child with a sister on either side of me, and I grew up with a close-knit family on the side of a Welsh mountain. Until the age of around ten years old, being ill never really featured in my life, other than frequent bouts of tonsillitis with similarly frequent courses of antibiotics. But things changed for me as I transitioned into adolescence.

Introduction

At first, I hardly even noticed psoriasis and it's only in retrospect that I can recall how it started; I fell in the school playground while running around with my friends and grazed my lower arms. Grazed knees and elbows were a normal part of my childhood, so this was nothing exceptional. It formed into a scab pretty quickly but strangely, the skin didn't heal. It just scabbed up, flaked off and scabbed up again. My parents were puzzled at how long the wound was taking to heal, but I didn't really think too much about it. My Mum kept putting new dressings on, occasionally the skin split and wept and eventually, after several weeks, it healed.

A few months later, I developed a patch of flaky skin on my scalp which I would pick at only to find a day later, it had reformed into a thick scab. I have a clear memory of standing in my Nan's front room with everyone looking at my scalp and none having a clue what it could be. Again, I don't remember being at all worried and just like my arms, eventually it went. I also had flaky skin in my belly button, but I didn't bother telling anyone about this. It itched like crazy and when I finally got to scratch it, a thick scab would peel off and give me a little relief from the itching. The skin underneath was red and smooth. Like the patch on my elbow and scalp, within hours, the scab had reformed. It didn't worry me at the time, but psoriasis in my belly button was to be an almost permanent feature of the next thirty years of my life.

By the age of 13, things had become a lot worse. I had red flaking skin on my eyelids and my eyebrows and large flaking plaques on my arms and legs. By now I was worried. It was very visible despite my best efforts to conceal it. In class, one of the boys loudly announced that I had eyebrow dandruff, much to the amusement of everyone, and I was mortified. Pretty soon after this, I was covered in thick plaques. There wasn't a place on my body that wasn't affected. I wore my hair with a thick fringe to hide the plaques on my forehead, but there was less I could do to disguise the ones on my eyelids and neck. My arms and legs were covered. I left piles of flaking skin wherever I went. My skin was so dry that it split and bled. At the end of the day, my clothes would have stuck to my skin, and I would have to peel them away, reopening the wound in the process.

I was eventually diagnosed with psoriasis at our local hospital. It was a word I'd never heard before, and I expected it to be like all my previous illnesses: I would get diagnosed, I would be given the right treatment and I would get rid of it. I took the diagnosis with relief. Now we knew what it was and I could do something about it. But this was not to be the case.

The next five or so years involved regular hospital visits, many different creams and ointments and every alternative treatment I could access. And nothing worked for long. Nothing. Eventually, a doctor told me that I now had to think of myself as someone with psoriasis in exactly the same way I thought of myself as someone with brown hair. It was not what I wanted to hear.

My skin got worse and worse, nothing seemed to help and hiding away became a way of life for me. I covered up as much as I could, avoided activities where I would have to undress, tried not to look at my reflection and wore long sleeves and trousers. I felt so ashamed of the way I looked, and though day to day I got on with life, I was always fearful of being found out to be the hideous creature I was under my clothes. When people asked me how I was doing, I smiled brightly and said 'fine' and hoped they couldn't tell how I really felt. I got very good at ignoring it. The trouble with hiding away and avoiding situations is that it isn't always under your control, and at times when I felt exposed like a school trip away or PE lessons, I had no strategy for coping and instead became anxious and miserable.

At the age of 18, I left home to study psychology at university. I'd always been interested in people, the mind and behaviour and this was the start of my career as a psychologist. As a new undergraduate, on top of dealing with leaving home and beginning student life, I had to deal with my skin. I'd worked all summer to save for a two-week holiday in Greece, and the healing power of the Mediterranean sun meant I arrived at university with almost clear skin. But as always, it didn't take long for things to deteriorate. The new doctor I registered with referred me for phototherapy alongside coal tar baths and an ointment that stained my skin and clothes, and to my shame, the bathtub in our communal halls of residence. No amount of scrubbing removed the blackened rings around the bathtub, and the smell of coal tar permeated throughout the corridors of my halls of residence. When people complained about the smell and the stains, I kept my eyes down and hoped they wouldn't find out it was me.

While my friends were studying and socialising, I would make the regular trip to the local hospital where I would have to completely undress, mortifying for a shy 18-year-old, and lie under a canopy of UVB lights which was lowered into place by rope and pulley by a physiotherapist with a stopwatch. She would start the timer and when it pinged, would call out for me to turn over from my front to expose my back to the rays, like a sausage on a barbecue. It worked and by the end of my first year of university, I was tanned all over and my skin was pretty clear. It was miraculous and I finally had the smooth skin I'd only been able to dream of.

However, as soon as the phototherapy treatment stopped, the psoriasis started to come back. Slowly at first, a few small spots here and there but then there would be a few more and I would watch my skin anxiously. At night, lying in bed, I would run my hand over my limbs in the dark feeling the new bumps and flakes with dismay. My body was a frightening and ever-changing landscape. I felt as though it betrayed me and the person I wanted to be.

This has been the pattern of my life ever since. Short-lived success with varied treatments and then anxious watching and monitoring as new plaques emerge and spread. If like me, you've had psoriasis for a long time, you will recognise the constant monitoring, the ever-changing severity, the new treatments, the hope and the disappointment.

All the while, my love of psychology grew, and I knew I wanted to pursue a career helping people manage psychological difficulties and mental health problems. After graduating, I moved to London and worked as an assistant psychologist in a team looking after people with respiratory diseases like asthma and chronic obstructive pulmonary disease (COPD). The consultant in charge of our department was revolutionary at the time and could see the complex links between physical health and emotional well-being. He employed a team of psychologists to study the relationship between physical symptoms and quality of life and, as someone who had lived uncomfortably with a skin disease by this time for over a decade, this made complete sense to me. I didn't look back and went on to complete my PhD, studying quality of life in people who have heart failure. Then, wanting to have more of an impact on people's lives, I trained as a clinical psychologist and have specialised in supporting people who live with chronic illness ever since.

Living with psoriasis

Around 1 million people in the United Kingdom and 7.5 million people in the United States have a diagnosis of psoriasis, making it a fairly common condition. Rates vary across the world; Norway has the highest prevalence with 2% of the population diagnosed and East Asia has the lowest prevalence at 0.12%. According to the Global Psoriasis Atlas, more than 60 million people across the world live with psoriasis (see the Resource section at the end of the book for more details about Global Psoriasis Atlas).

Most people will think of psoriasis as a skin condition, but in recent years scientists have come to understand that it's an immune-mediated condition affecting many systems in the body. That means the immune system isn't working properly, resulting in inflammation. On lighter skin, psoriasis appears as plaques, usually red and raised, and these are formed by the overproduction of skin cells. On darker skin, the plaques can look purple or grey which is not commonly represented in the media and may lead to misdiagnosis and underreporting in black people (Alexis & Blackcloud, 2014).

There are different forms of psoriasis, the most common of which is chronic plaque psoriasis, where the lesions are typically round in shape, a few centimetres in diameter, raised and covered in a silvery scale. In chronic plaque psoriasis, the most common areas of the body to be affected include the scalp, knees, elbows, belly button and genitals. However, plaques can occur on any area of the body, for example in the ears, on the eyelids, on the palms of hands and on the soles of the feet.

Other forms of psoriasis include guttate psoriasis, in which the lesions are small, drop-like and often extensive, and pustular psoriasis, in which the lesions are characterised by pus-filled bumps or pustules. Erythrodermic psoriasis is a rarer form of the condition in which the whole body is affected by erythroderma (reddening of the skin) and scaling. Erythrodermic psoriasis requires emergency treatment and can lead to death if left untreated.

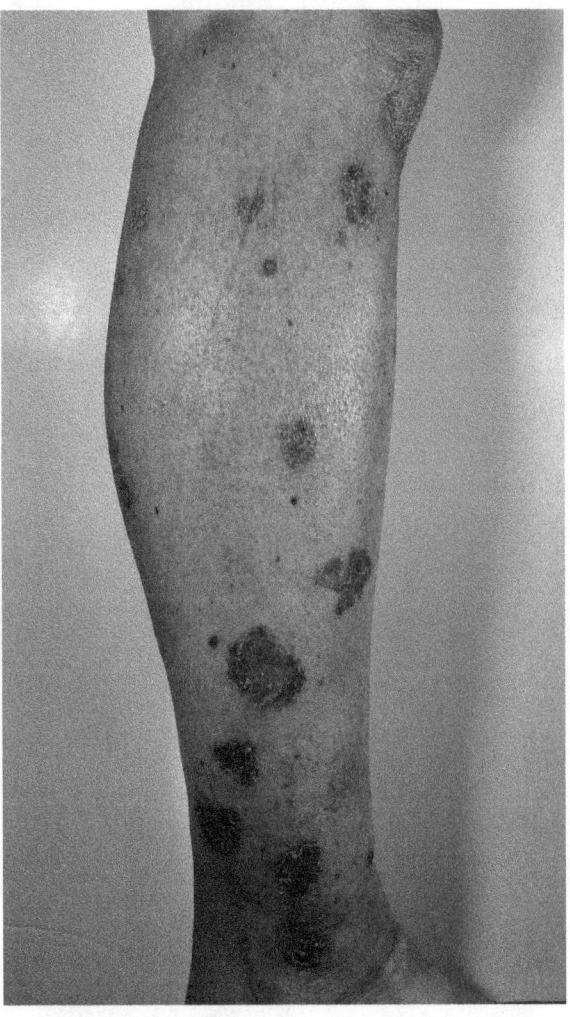

1. Plaque psoriasis on the lower leg

COPING WITH PSORIASIS

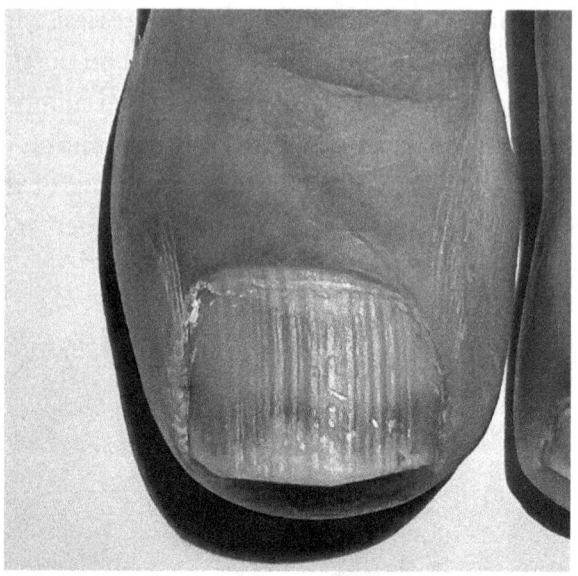

2. Psoriasis of the toenail

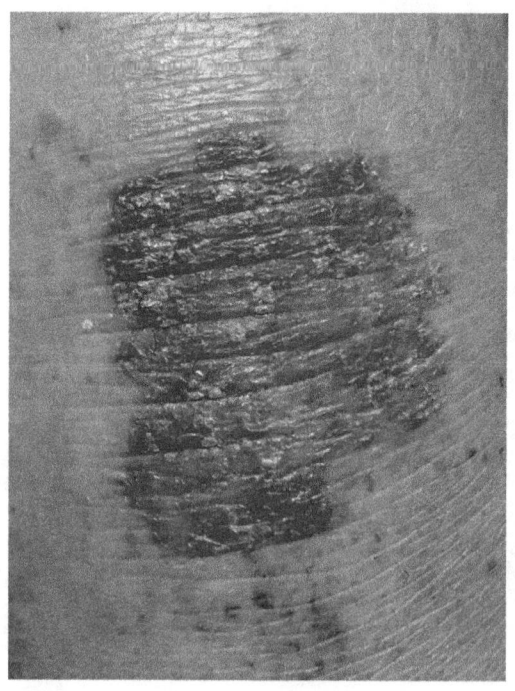

3. A typical plaque

In addition to the skin lesions, fingernails and toenails may be affected by pitting, discolouration and separation from the nail bed. Around 30% of people also develop PsA, which is inflammation of the joints, tendons and ligaments. While never formally diagnosed with PsA, I've had periods where the joints in my fingers, wrists, elbows and toes ache and swell, mostly in the evenings. Luckily, these seem to pass after a few weeks and then I can go for long periods without any joint pain at all. For some people though, PsA can be very disabling and affect mobility and independence.

Psoriasis is also characterised by the Koebner phenomenon, with lesions occurring where there has been skin trauma or injury, such as a cut, an injection site or a burn. This means if you fall and injure your skin, it's very likely to turn into psoriasis. After having my ears pierced, the holes in my earlobes were covered with psoriasis for decades. In my twenties, I had my belly button pierced and that turned into a patch of psoriasis that regularly flaked and became infected until I gave up and removed it.

For most people, the severity of psoriasis is rarely static. Individuals are likely to cycle between differing levels of severity throughout their lifetime. Many individuals with psoriasis experience 'spontaneous' remissions and flare-ups throughout the course of their condition.

Physiological mechanisms resulting in psoriasis are complex. In certain patches, the normal process of skin cell renewal speeds up. In an average individual, normal skin turnover takes 27 days, which means that it's not at all noticeable. In psoriatic lesions, this process takes only three or four days. The skin cells renew so fast that they don't shed so effectively and start to build up on the surface of the skin. Alongside the accelerated skin renewal, there are alterations in the shape of the blood capillaries and increased delivery of blood to the skin surface. These changes result in red, scaly patches of skin.

We don't know why some people develop psoriasis, though there is evidence that it can be triggered by several factors such as trauma to the skin, infection or certain medication. It is thought to have a hereditary element with approximately 30% of people with psoriasis having a family member also with psoriasis (Krueger et al., 1994). There is also some evidence of immune system involvement with T cells, which are involved in the normal immune response, playing a significant role. Dermatologists believe genetics and the environment are involved in the development and maintenance of psoriasis. Psoriasis is not contagious.

Psoriasis is so much more than a skin disease. It's easy to tell yourself that you should be able to cope with psoriasis, that it's just a skin disease, but as you read through this book, you'll see how living with a constant but ever-changing skin condition can slowly erode away your confidence and self-esteem. Bit by bit, it can change the way you deal with life, with other people and it changes the way you cope with a crisis. This can make you vulnerable to developing mental health struggles.

I think of the plaques of psoriatic skin as only the tip of the iceberg; the visible symptoms that are obvious to others. But below the surface is a vast body of invisible scars and symptoms: shame, pain, sleep problems, low confidence and anxiety to name a few of the hidden impacts. It's absolutely possible to have psoriasis and experience only a few or none of the impacts under the water, but chances are, like me, it will have affected you (Figure 1.1).

Living with psoriasis has an enormous psychological impact and many people struggle. John Updike, the American author, wrote movingly about his own experience of psoriasis and how it impacted his life and sense of self. In an article for the *New Yorker* magazine, he described psoriasis as being, 'the sense of another presence co-occupying your body and singling you out from the happy herds of normal mankind' (Updike, 1985). Musician Cyndi Lauper has described psoriasis as 'swallowing me up'. You're not alone in dealing with this.

It's taken me a long time to build up the courage to write this book. I've always been especially good at hiding my skin and I never really wanted people to know me as someone with psoriasis. Though my close friends and family are aware, I have always hidden my skin from

Introduction

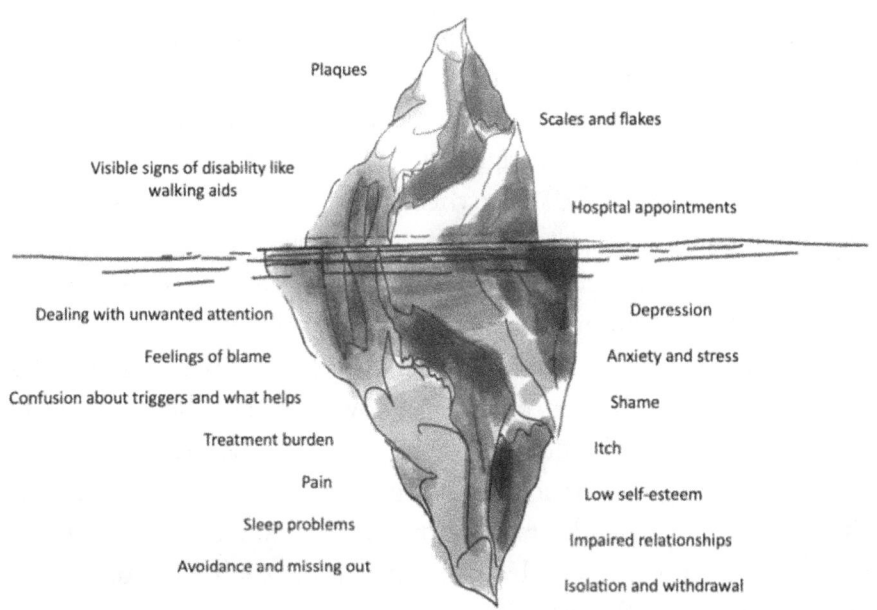

FIGURE 1.1 Psoriasis iceberg

them. At times when it's bad, I even hide it from myself by avoiding my reflection in the mirror. Throughout my childhood and adolescence, I learnt to feel ashamed of the way I looked, and I became fearful of how people would view me if they knew how I looked beneath my clothes. This has not only had a big impact on the things I've done in my life, the choices I've made, the activities I've avoided and the opportunities I've missed, but it's also affected the way I cope with difficulties and how I manage problems in my life.

I'm a clinical psychologist, which means that perhaps more than most, I'm aware of the way psoriasis affects me emotionally and how it's had a deep-seated impact on my development. I want to use these insights in the hope that it will help others to understand the impact it's had on them, their lives and relationships, as well as the things that can help.

Over the years, I've worked with people with varied health conditions including cleft lip and palate, kidney failure and respiratory disease; along the way, I've learnt a lot about coping with illness. I've worked alongside brilliant psychologists and physicians, and I've met patients who have inspired and humbled me. All this experience has helped me understand how psoriasis affects me and how best to cope with it. I don't always get it right, and I've learnt that it's very normal to have times when it feels overwhelming. I live with a very challenging health condition, and I wouldn't be human if I didn't struggle at times. I continue to study and learn. I continue to wish and hope for a cure, but like everything else, my psoriasis continues too.

I've reached a point in my life where I feel much braver about telling the world about my struggles and how I manage them. I want to share with you what I've learnt about living with psoriasis in the hope that it will help you cope too. By bringing you research evidence, psychological theories, understanding and strategies, I want to empower you with the knowledge to learn to cope and live a life full of joy and meaning, in spite of psoriasis.

2   Psoriasis and depression

Living with psoriasis often makes me feel down and unhappy. There have been a few occasions in my life when this felt much worse, and I suspect I was clinically depressed. There was a time in my late twenties when I was feeling at a particularly low point in my life. I had just lost my beloved grandmother, I was in the final stressful stages of my PhD, thinking about the next step in my career, and on top of everything else, I was covered head to toe in psoriasis. I felt sore and flaking all the time and was trying my best with topical treatments that were burdensome and not especially effective. My ears were blocked with plaques and skin, and that affected my hearing and balance. Around the same time, a doctor told me there was a very real risk of me losing my hair because of the thickened plaques on my scalp.

After years of living with psoriasis, hiding away both my skin and my feelings had all become too much. I took down the mirrors in my home, save for a small bathroom mirror at head height. I felt if I didn't have to look at my reflection, I would feel better about myself. It didn't really help, and I began to feel worse about the way I looked. The plaques of psoriasis increased in size and number, and I started to fear I wouldn't have any normal skin left. As my mood sank, I found it harder to socialise and started to refuse invitations. I lost my appetite, my sleep was all over the place and I would lie in bed at night, scratching at my skin. I began to feel as though there was a black cloud hanging over my head.

I'm not alone in having periods of depression in relation to my skin. There's a lot of evidence to demonstrate a strong link between depression and psoriasis.

Links between psoriasis and depression

In the general population, approximately 10% of people have experienced depression at some point in their lives. It's so common that some people have gone as far as to describe it as the common cold of mental health problems.

Yet there is evidence of greater prevalence in people with psoriasis. It is difficult to estimate the exact number of people with psoriasis who are depressed, because rates vary from study to study depending on how depression was measured. Reported rates range from 9%, which is similar to rates in the general population, to around 20% (Mathew & Chandran, 2020a), 55% (Fabrazzo et al., 2022) and even 60% (Esposito et al., 2006).

Despite the high prevalence found in some studies, it's clear that just because you have psoriasis, it doesn't mean that it's inevitable that you'll become depressed. Even in those research studies that found high rates of depression, there was a large group of people with psoriasis who weren't experiencing depression. So, it's important to remember that a significant number of people won't feel depressed.

What this research does mean though, is that having psoriasis is going to make you more vulnerable to becoming depressed. For me, that seems to be especially the case if the plaques occur in places that are difficult to hide or when the condition is more severe. I remember a time when I had prominent psoriasis on my fingernails and the backs of my hands and wrists, and I cringed inside every time I paid at a till and had to hand over money. Despite my best efforts to hide psoriasis from myself and the world, it was hard to ignore when I saw it all the time. In fact, people with psoriasis on their hands and fingernails report being more distressed than those with psoriasis on the face and scalp, even when their psoriasis is mild (Ohata et al., 2019, Hawro et al., 2017).

Is this clinical depression?

People often describe themselves as depressed as a shorthand way to describe feeling unhappy or blue. However, I know from my experience that clinical depression is more than this. Unlike depression, feelings of sadness or low mood from time to time are part of a range of normal human emotions. Everyone feels this way, and there are times when it's a very appropriate reaction to a difficult life event. Clinical depression is different because of the intensity and range of feelings as well as the length of time it lasts.

Depression is diagnosed when people experience a cluster of symptoms shown in Figure 2.1.

Some of these symptoms also overlap with psoriasis and psoriatic arthritis (PsA); for example, aches and pains, sleep problems, changes in energy and wanting to isolate yourself may all be physical symptoms of the condition. It can be tricky to work out if what you're feeling is due to a flare in your psoriasis symptoms, because you're depressed or both.

People don't become depressed overnight. Like a lot of people, my mood started to dip slowly so that it was difficult for me to tell just how low I'd become. It happens little by little and you get used to feeling low, having no energy and not wanting to engage with the world.

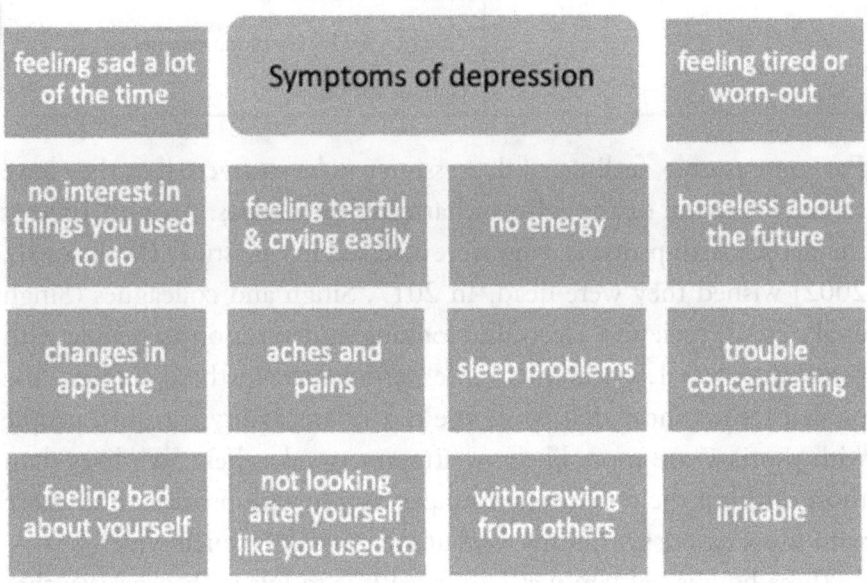

FIGURE 2.1 Symptoms of depression

It becomes your new norm. It's often so difficult to tell when you're feeling depressed that for a lot of people, it's only diagnosed when people finally reach out for help, prompted by not being able to carry on with daily life or to continue functioning at work.

Many mental health clinicians use a medical coding system, the International Classification of Diseases (ICD-10), to diagnose someone with depression. The ICD-10 criteria for clinical depression is when at least one of the key symptoms has been present most days, most of the time for at least two weeks, alongside at least two of the associated symptoms. The number of associated symptoms present determines the severity of the depression.

Key symptoms	Associated symptoms
Persistent sadness or low mood	Disturbed sleep
Loss of interest or pleasure	Poor concentration or indecisiveness
Fatigue or low energy	Low self-confidence
	Poor or increased appetite
	Suicidal thoughts or acts
	Agitation or slowing of movements
	Guilt or self-blame

For some people, feelings of depression can be so severe that they have suicidal ideation or thoughts of harming themselves. Around 10% of the people with psoriasis who were assessed in one study (Weiss et al., 2002) wished they were dead. In 2017, Singh and colleagues (Singh et al., 2017) reviewed 18 studies looking at depression in people with psoriasis. Over 1.5 million people participated in these studies. The pooled results show that while the risk of suicidality was low, people with psoriasis are more likely to attempt to take their own lives than those without the condition. Younger people with psoriasis and those with more severe symptoms were at greater risk of suicidality.

These figures tell you just how hard it is to live with psoriasis; that life can feel so challenging that at times many people wish it would all just stop. I know for myself it has never been that I didn't want to live but more that I was exhausted from struggling with my skin and feeling like there was no way to get control. It felt like a constant battle where I didn't know the rules. I wasn't exactly sure who I was fighting, but I knew I was losing horribly. I have had times in my life when I would go to bed at night and think it would all be so much easier if I didn't wake up in the morning. In the Appendix, there is advice on when and where to seek help and what to do if you're having thoughts of suicide (see Mental health concerns).

Developing depression when you have psoriasis

It's believed that in the general population people become depressed due to a complex mix of biological, social and psychological factors. As you read through this book, you'll begin to understand why you're much more likely to be depressed when you have psoriasis. There's not just one reason but a complex pattern of stresses that increase your risk of feeling depressed, like experiences of discrimination and bullying, relationship difficulties and feelings of shame and low self-worth. All of these will be addressed in later chapters.

In addition to life stresses and challenges, some scientists believe there is a genetic predisposition to depression and that you're more likely to be depressed if one of your parents has also been depressed. The biomedical picture of psoriasis is even more complex.

There's emerging evidence that people with psoriasis may be at more risk of developing depression, not solely due to the impact of psoriasis on life, but because of the biological mechanisms linked with the development of both conditions. For example, low vitamin D3 and inflammatory disease processes appear to be factors common to the development of both depression and psoriasis (Sahi et al., 2020).

Similarly, another research study found that inflammation arising from elevated cytokines, the proteins involved in inflammation, may also cause physiological and biochemical changes that directly impact on mood disorders including depression (Koo et al., 2017).

The role of inflammatory processes involved in both depression and anxiety is very interesting. It's a complex science, but what it essentially means is the biological factors predetermining you to develop psoriasis may also mean you are predetermined to develop depression. There's some evidence in people with PsA to suggest that treatments which target the inflammatory processes in PsA are also more likely to improve symptoms of depression than the more conventional antidepressant treatments (Mathew & Chandran, 2020b).

There's also interesting research being conducted into the impact of the gut microbiome on psoriasis, and also mood and depression. The gut microbiome is the name given to the millions of microorganisms living in your gut. These cells are responsible for stimulating the immune system, breaking down food, and producing vitamins and biochemicals the body needs to function well. Everyone has an entirely unique make-up of cells determined by numerous factors such as diet, lifestyle and medications. Fermented foods such as kimchi are said to encourage healthy, diverse bacteria, whereas diets which are heavily processed food based are more likely to lead to a less diverse microbiome.

Scientists are beginning to understand the important role of the microbiome in emotional well-being, as it appears to play an important role in producing serotonin, one of the neurotransmitters involved in lifting and stabilising mood. There is some evidence to suggest that depression can be improved by taking probiotics and changing diet alone (Huang et al., 2016). At the same time, scientists are beginning to understand the role of the gut in psoriasis, though many experts have talked about 'leaky gut syndrome' and psoriasis for decades (Ely, 2018; Sikora et al., 2020).

As you can see, it's very complex and it is likely that depression relating to psoriasis results from a myriad of factors. With much of this research still in its infancy, we're only just beginning to understand the implications.

One of the most difficult things about living with depression is the negative downward spiral that's so hard to lift yourself from. When someone feels depressed, it not only affects the way they feel but also how they start to think and behave. These changes then make it more likely that the feelings of depression will persist.

In terms of thinking, if you feel depressed, you may notice that your thoughts have also become quite negative. It's normal to be thinking most of the time. We all have a running commentary going on in our heads whatever we're doing. Even as you're reading this book, I expect you'll have other thought processes going on at the same time as you're reading the words. You might be thinking about the book, like 'I'm going to see if I can find that reference to read more', or it may even be very mundane things not related to the text at all, such as, 'I'll need to put this book down in a minute to start cooking dinner'.

When depressed, people's thought commentary tends to become overly negative. What this means is that if you're depressed, you'll probably start to think about the world around you and things that are happening in an overly negative way, and without really even noticing that's happened. For example, if you're late to a meeting because the traffic's busy, you may think, 'Nothing ever goes right for me. I should have left earlier. I never plan anything well. There's really no point in trying'. The person in a car behind you, in exactly the same traffic with exactly the same delay, might be thinking instead, 'What a pain. I wonder if there was an accident. I'm so glad I wasn't caught up in that'. It's easy to see how the very same traffic jam can end up with one person feeling bad about themselves and the other person, frustrated but not blaming themselves at all. When you get to Chapters 11 and 12, there's information on the way psoriasis impacts thinking and ways to manage negative thought patterns.

When it comes to psoriasis, the negative thinking and hopelessness that go hand in hand with feelings of depression mean that you start to believe there's no solution, no treatments will ever work and nothing you can do will make a difference. If you start to tell yourself this, you are not only going to feel more depressed but also this hopelessness means you are far less likely to adhere to your treatments. It may seem like too much effort for too little return. These thoughts may also start to have implications on your lifestyle; you may drink more, start to eat more junk food and do less exercise.

When people become depressed, their behaviour also changes. It's common for people to stop doing the things they enjoy and spending time with the people they love, isolating themselves from the world and others. Life can become lonely and unsatisfying, and if you already feel ashamed of the way you look because of psoriasis, isolation can add to the feelings of low self-worth. It's easy to see how this behaviour can add to the downward spiral (Figure 2.2).

Treating depression

If you've read through the list of symptoms of depression and you recognise some of the ways of thinking and behaving, then you might be depressed. If this is the case, then it's important for you to know two things. First, you're not depressed because you're weak, a failure or defective, and there's no reason to feel ashamed. Depression affects all sorts of people from all walks of life, including celebrities and millionaires. Psoriasis is a difficult condition to live with, and it's not surprising that many people feel depressed at times, myself included.

Second, it's important for you to know that depression is treatable with talking therapy or with antidepressant medication, or a combination of both, so don't give up hope. That's not to say it's easy to just pull yourself together and snap out of depression. If it was that simple, I'm sure most people would do that straightaway. With the right help, most people can learn to manage their feelings of depression.

In the UK, the National Institute for Health and Care Excellence (NICE) has published guidelines for the treatment of depression in people with chronic illness. These guidelines are written by a panel of experts based on the latest research evidence. For mild-to-moderate depression, they recommend psychosocial interventions like peer support, psychological interventions and medication. Depending on the severity of the depression, psychological treatments include cognitive behavioural therapy (CBT) in the form of either self-help,

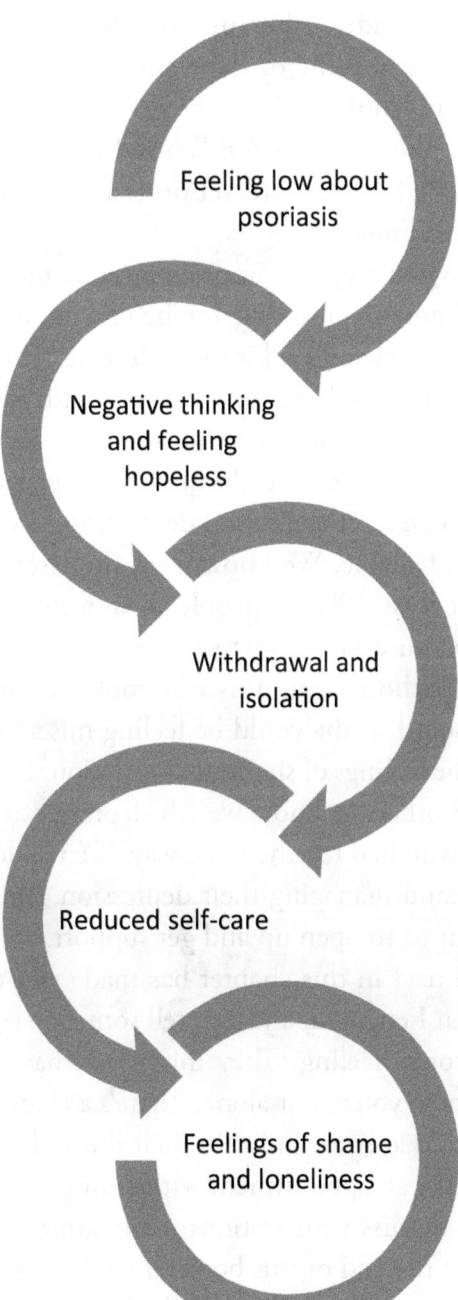

FIGURE 2.2 Negative spiral of depression in psoriasis

group-based or individual therapy. The NICE guidelines for the treatment and management of depression in adults recommend a wider range of psychological interventions alongside antidepressant medication. These include CBT, mindfulness and Interpersonal Psychotherapy (IPT). These interventions and strategies will be discussed later in this book.

One of the biggest steps to improving your mood is recognising you're depressed and then asking for help. Lots of people who are depressed feel ashamed and find it difficult to tell people. As a clinical psychologist, I frequently have conversations with my clients encouraging them to be open to people about their own depression. In general, people don't find it easy to do that. Most people, even those in therapy, tend to hide their feelings of depression, which only perpetuates the feelings of shame. We know from the research evidence that there must be at least 10% of people in our communities who are depressed, but because of the secrecy, we don't know who they are. It's very likely that those around us who look like they're leading the perfect lives on social media could be feeling miserable on the inside. This all adds to the feelings of shame and isolation. If only we all talked about it, allowed others to know we felt depressed then we could see those around us who had felt the same way. We would also know who was getting help and managing their depression. This would make it so much easier for us to open up and get support.

If what you've read in this chapter has made you think you might be depressed, then I encourage you to tell someone you love and trust about the way you're feeling. They might not have all the answers, but it helps to know you're not alone. There's a chance they may even have been depressed at some point in their life and know exactly how you're feeling. Make an appointment with your general practitioner or dermatologist to discuss your options for treatment and have a look at the resources at the end of this book. If you're finding it difficult to tell what's symptoms of psoriasis and what's symptoms of depression, talking to a clinician can help you unpick the symptoms and work out what's going on.

Changing your behaviour can also help. We know that when people become depressed, they stop doing the things that bring them happiness and a sense of purpose. This starts a cycle of inactivity leading to low mood leading to inactivity and so on. People tend to carry on with the essential tasks of life, like getting dressed and going to work, but sometimes when depression is severe, even those things stop. Psychologists call purposely scheduling activity which brings feelings of pleasure and mastery 'behavioural reactivation' and there's good evidence that it helps with depression.

> **Try this**
>
> You could start behavioural reactivation by introducing something simple that you used to enjoy, like a walk in the park, and then think about restarting or taking up activities or hobbies. Try to make sure that every day you do something that brings you a sense of mastery and pleasure, schedule it in your diary so you know what you're going to do and when. It's hard to start increasing your activity when you don't feel like it, but the trick is to just start anyway. Eventually, your days will begin to feel more pleasurable and more meaningful.

As I mentioned at the beginning of this chapter, psoriasis is more than a skin disease. The following chapters will help you to understand the iceberg under the surface of the water; the feelings of shame, blame, low self-esteem, poor confidence, which are so familiar to those of us with the condition. This book will help you recognise the stresses associated with living with psoriasis. As a clinical psychologist who works with people with health conditions, I'm confident the strategies in this book will not only help you to understand how psoriasis can affect you but also give you ways to deal with the challenges, and in doing so, help to improve your mood.

Summary

- Many people with psoriasis feel depressed. This is because it can be a very hard condition to live with.
- Depression affects how you feel, the way you think and what you do or don't do.
- Depression can become a negative spiral with negative thinking and withdrawing from friends and the world, leading to more feelings of depression.
- You might feel ashamed about being depressed, but remember it's very common, and the chances are that those around you understand exactly how you're feeling, so tell someone you trust.
- Depression is treatable. There are antidepressant medications and psychological therapies which can help.

Top tips

- It can be hard to tell if you're depressed if you've been feeling low for some time.
- Try to think about what's changed in your life: Have you stopped seeing friends? Have you stopped enjoying your hobbies? Have you lost interest in the way you look? These may be signs you have become depressed.
- If you think you're depressed, tell someone.
- Remember, this is not your fault.

3 Psoriasis and stress

If you have psoriasis, you won't be a stranger to the idea that it is linked to stress. Many people with psoriasis commonly associate flares in their condition with life stresses. Some people believe that a stressful event was the thing that triggered their psoriasis to develop in the first place.

Besides people's own anecdotal evidence, there's some clinical evidence to suggest a link. However, much of this evidence is retrospective, asking people to think back to whether a stressful time or event might have preceded the flare-up in their psoriasis. This type of research depends on people's ability to recall accurately and objectively the patterns of flare-ups. Despite flaws in the use of retrospective evidence, researchers have determined a link exists between psoriasis and stress in this way. However, when you look at the range of these types of studies, the findings are mixed. In some research studies, people with psoriasis believed stress was related to their condition while others found no relationship (Snast et al., 2018). What's interesting is that people were less likely to notice a link in the older studies conducted in the 1970s and much more likely to report a link in studies published after the 1990s (Berg et al., 2008). This may relate to the increasing popularity of the theory that stress causes psoriasis.

A study of people hospitalised with psoriasis asked them to complete a questionnaire measuring stressful life events in the past year. They found there was no difference in the frequency of stressful life events in the year before the admission than there was in their control group made up of people with other skin conditions (Picardi et al., 2005). This supports other studies which also didn't find an excess of stressful life events before an exacerbation leading to a hospital admission.

There have been a few attempts to conduct prospective studies, which means studying people over time and asking them to keep diaries where they rate their daily stress levels and symptoms of psoriasis.

This way, you can track whether stress precedes a worsening of symptoms. One such study conducted in Sweden (Berg et al., 2008) asked nine women with stable psoriasis to give daily estimates of both psoriasis and stress over varying periods of time. The assumption was that if there was a connection between stress and psoriasis, the exacerbation would occur between one and three weeks after the stressors occurred. Therefore, the women were asked to stop recording when their skin was 25% more severe than it had been at the start of the study. At the start of the study, all women believed their psoriasis was stress-dependent. At the end of the study, no clear pattern had emerged despite varying levels of stress over the course of the study. Only one person had elevated stress levels 13 days before her psoriasis worsened. For the majority, there was no connection between stress and worsening psoriasis at all. However, in two individuals, their stress levels rose significantly *after* the worsening of psoriasis symptoms. It's worth bearing in mind that the sample studied was small and because of that, it's difficult to draw firm conclusions.

When I was training to be a clinical psychologist, I was required to conduct and write up a research study as part of my doctorate. I jumped at the opportunity to look at the psychological impact of psoriasis and asked ten people to keep diaries for four weeks of their psoriasis and stress. Like the Swedish study, there was no clear pattern between the two. What was interesting to me was at the start of the study, I asked people to report what factors were responsible for them developing psoriasis. What emerged was that if someone believed stress was responsible, they were much more likely to feel depressed and anxious than if they believed there were other possible causes such as genetics or the environmental factors (O'Leary et al., 2004). It made me wonder whether it's a good thing that our dermatologists, doctors, family and friends often ask about stress, feeding the current popular narrative that the two are inextricably linked. I suspect it contributes to our feelings of shame and self-blame. There have been many times when I've told myself that having psoriasis is my fault and that I'm doing something wrong; telling myself that I'm someone who gets stressed too easily or too much may become just another stick with which to beat myself.

As a psychologist who is trained in understanding anxiety and spends a lot of time helping people monitor and manage their own stress, I've been in a good position to look for links between stress in my life and my condition. I've never really noticed a clear pattern. Like everyone, I experience periods of stress and certain things make me anxious, but I'm unsure how this relates to my skin. Despite this, just about every time I visit a doctor with a flare-up, I'm asked if I feel stressed or whether I've been having a particularly stressful time. At that point, after waiting for a hospital appointment and being concerned about whether the next round of phototherapy would work, I am feeling a certain amount of stress. I don't know what came first. Similarly, friends and family will tut sympathetically if they catch a glimpse of my skin and ask how my stress levels are, assuming that because they see one, the other must be close behind. It's made me very conscious of minimising stress in my life, just in case it does make my skin worse, to the point where I won't watch a scary or tense movie which might send my heart racing. It sounds ridiculous as I type this but is true.

The role of stress in psoriasis

Despite the lack of clear-cut evidence confirming that stress triggers or causes psoriasis to flare, there are numerous theories explaining the role of stress in psoriasis. Importantly, there does appear to be a relationship between inflammation and stress. Stress causes the body to produce cortisol, a steroid hormone to help the body deal with the physiological demands of stress. One of its functions is to suppress inflammation, but prolonged stress and over-production of cortisol mean that over time, the body becomes less sensitive to cortisol. It ceases to reduce inflammation as effectively.

It's also clear that living with psoriasis is, in itself, stressful. We know that when people feel under stress, this has an impact on well-being and behaviour. Stress can affect sleep patterns, diet and eating habits, alcohol consumption and many other health-related behaviours. People living with significant amounts of stress may find it more difficult to prioritise their treatments and find time to apply messy ointments twice a day. They may be so overwhelmed they forget to take their tablets and miss appointments. There's evidence that anxiety about psoriasis is stable and doesn't improve even when the skin does. Even when in remission, people scan for new patches (Jowett & Ryan, 1985). The complexity of this picture makes it almost impossible to figure out which came first, the stress or the psoriasis (Figure 3.1).

In his book about skin and his own experience of psoriasis, Sergio del Molino (del Molino Sergio, 2021) describes writer Vladimir Nabakov's letters to his wife during a particularly bad flare. At the same time as this was happening, Nabakov was working away from home and had started an affair, leading many historians to conclude that the stress of being unfaithful came first and was responsible for his worsening skin. His psoriasis 'was an expression of his distress … and the idea that this bout was caused by the tension and bad conscience of his love'. Del Molino points out, though, that as soon as Nabakov began phototherapy and his skin started to clear, his letters took an entirely different tone. The affair, and presumed guilt and stress, was ongoing but now, his psoriasis had cleared. This led del Molino to conclude that the symptoms of psoriasis caused the stress and not the other way around. This fits with his own experience of psoriasis; 'that it isn't the

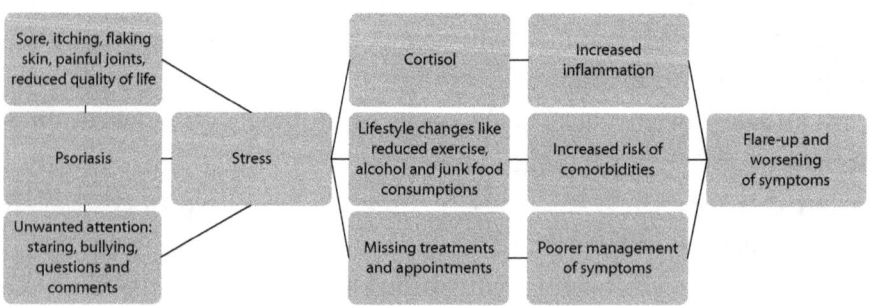

FIGURE 3.1 Proposed pathway between stress and psoriasis

person's state of mind that aggravates the psoriasis ... but that the psoriasis itself that embitters a person's nature'.

There is some evidence that interventions designed to improve stress levels also improve psoriasis (Rousset & Halioua, 2018). One study (Kabat-Zinn et al., 1998) took 37 people about to start phototherapy (UVB and PUVA) for their psoriasis. Half of the group went ahead with treatment as usual. The other half listened to a mindfulness recording while they were in the phototherapy machine. The results showed that those who did mindfulness at the same time as phototherapy cleared significantly faster than those in the control condition.

More recent research has also shown a benefit of meditation in psoriasis. A review of six studies (Bartholomew et al., 2022) where people were randomised to a control group or to do meditation found that in five of these, severity of psoriasis improved significantly more in the meditation group after 8 or 12 weeks of practice. Two of these studies also showed psychological improvements related to the meditation.

Stress is a normal human emotion

So far in this chapter, I've talked about stress like we all know what we're referring to; we know what it means to be under stress, to face stressful events, to feel stress. However, you may find it helpful to understand why we feel stress, what happens to our bodies when we're under stress and what we can do about it.

Stress can be taken to mean an emotional demand on an individual, as well as the emotional reaction to feeling under pressure or threat. In everyday life, people tend to use the terms stress and anxiety interchangeably, but anxiety refers to persistent or excessive worries even when there is no threat or external stressor present.

You'd be a very unusual person if you didn't ever experience stress. Stress is a normal human reaction and it's essential to our survival as a species. As humans, we come with a built-in alarm system to help us deal with threats and danger. Like all good alarm systems, it's very easily triggered. It would be no good raising a signal to react several minutes after a danger has presented itself or to miss a subtle sign that we're in danger. In order to survive, we need to be good at reacting and reacting quickly.

This sensitive alarm system was essential to our ancestors' survival, arguably more so than it is for us in modern times. It can help to imagine a human hundreds of years ago looking for food in the forest. Gathering food was a more dangerous activity for our ancestors than it is for us. They needed to be alert to a rustling bush or the howl of a wolf, and they would need to react quickly. If they didn't react, then there's a good chance they wouldn't make it home for dinner and you can see how over time, the gene for an easily triggered alarm system would be passed on through the generations. Those with a less sensitive alarm system were far less likely to be living long enough to successfully raise a family.

Our hunter-gatherer ancestors would hear a rustling bush in the depths of the forest and their bodies would react so they could deal with whatever was making that noise. That might mean fighting or it might mean running away, a response we call 'fight or flight'.

Even today, you can see how important it is for us to have an easily triggered alarm system. Dangers may be different now than they were for our ancestors, but we still need to be able to react appropriately. This means when faced with a threat, our bodies react automatically so we don't have to wonder why there is a lion rampaging through the corridor at work, we don't have to think through the hows or the whys or our options. We can just fight or flee and get to safety. Psychologists now also talk about the freeze response when the body becomes immobile in the face of danger.

Once the alarm has been triggered, our bodies react to danger in various ways to help us deal with it. Our breathing becomes rapid, our hearts beat faster to pump blood around our body and get our muscles primed for action. The extra oxygen can make us feel lightheaded or dizzy. Our livers release glucose for energy. We might feel the need to go to the toilet as we need to be as light as possible. We stop digesting our food, and this causes a dry mouth and can make us feel sick or experience butterflies in our stomachs. Our brain instructs our bodies to produce stress hormones such as adrenaline and cortisol. The front of our brain, the region for more complex thinking and planning, effectively shuts down. We don't need to be analysing the situation until we're in a place of safety.

All of this can feel unpleasant, but it makes perfect sense when there's a lion rampaging or a fire has broken out. Unfortunately, what happens in the modern world is that this response is triggered when there is no immediate danger. Simply remembering a threat from the past or worrying about a threat that might happen in the future can start the process and before we know it, we're in full fight or flight mode, with our hearts beating hard, sweating and feeling sick, but there's nothing to run away from or fight.

What can then happen is that those unpleasant feelings become the threat: 'What's happening to me?', 'This is horrible', 'Am I having a heart attack?', 'Can everyone tell I'm having a panic attack?' and then these thoughts keep it going longer.

Over time, you can become scared of this happening and so you start to avoid things and sometimes trigger a panic attack by worrying about having one. It can become a vicious cycle (Figure 3.2).

Adversity in childhood

In recent years, we've become aware of the impact of stress in childhood on people's mental and physical health in adulthood. Adversity in childhood results in repeated triggering of the fight or flight response which over time impacts neurological, immunological, hormonal and even brain development. There seems to be something about being in threat mode frequently during childhood that wires the brain to be prepared for danger, increasing tissue inflammation and resulting in long-term changes in immune response. This leads to tissue damage and long-term wear and tear on the body.

There's preliminary evidence that adults with psoriasis have experienced more childhood trauma, also known as Adverse Childhood Experiences (ACEs) than age and gender-matched controls

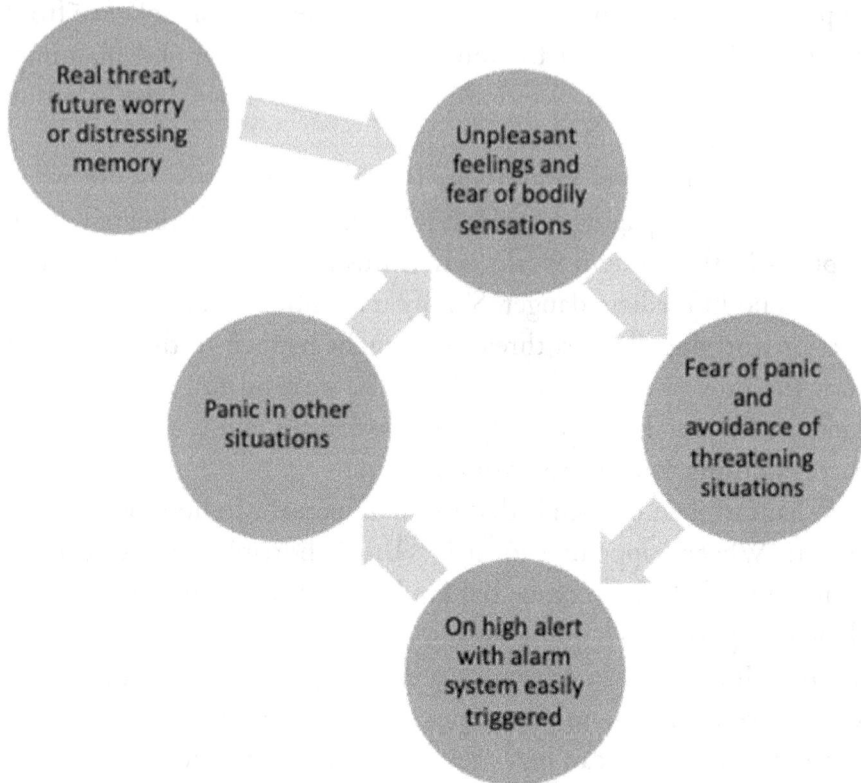

FIGURE 3.2 Vicious cycle of panic

(Akamine et al., 2021). The ACEs in this study included childhood abuse, neglect and household dysfunction.

There is a large body of research looking at the prevalence of ACEs in the general population and the impact of these in later life. We know that having a history of ACEs increases your risk of health-harming behaviours such as smoking, drinking or eating too much of the wrong stuff. You might think these lifestyle choices are responsible for the increased risks to health, but that's just not the case. After controlling for differences in lifestyle choices, there is convincing evidence that people who experience ACEs are at a much higher risk for many long-term health conditions like autoimmune disorders such as psoriasis, cancer, lung disease, heart disease and mental illness. They can even shorten your life by 20 years, and the more ACEs you have, the higher your risk. In one long-term study (Danese et al., 2007), childhood abuse was associated with elevated markers of infection and inflammation in blood samples 20 years later.

Psychological strategies for managing stress and anxiety

The fight or flight response and feeling stressed are both normal and important human reactions to adversity and life challenges. Even if I were 100% confident that stress is related to psoriasis, I would not be able to eliminate stress from my life in order to clear my skin. Similarly, I would not be able to stop my body from reacting and going into fight or flight mode if I were in a dangerous situation. The fight or flight response can be literally lifesaving, but it can also be helpful for situations that aren't life-threatening. If I have to give a presentation at a conference, I accept that I will feel nervous and anxious beforehand because it's important to do well, and the stress hormones my body produces will help me perform. Interestingly, if I'm in the queue for a rollercoaster, I get exactly the same feelings, but because I'm choosing to frighten myself in the name of fun, I don't pay too much attention to the butterflies and nervous energy and put it down to excitement. Reacting to stress and feeling anxious is part of being human.

Despite that, I don't want to be experiencing stress when I don't need to. I know that memories and worries about the future may trigger a stress reaction in my body, and I also know that increased levels of stress hormones aren't going to be helpful to any inflammation going on in my body. It also doesn't feel very nice to be stressed if you don't have to be.

Practising mindfulness

Because I don't want my body to be triggered all the time by my busy mind, I practise mindfulness meditation regularly. I don't do this thinking I'm going to clear up my psoriasis. Instead, I'm led by the overwhelming evidence which shows that mindfulness can have significant benefits not only on emotional well-being, improving both anxiety and depression, but it also has other benefits such as improved decision-making and stronger feelings of compassion for self and others. As described earlier in this chapter, mindfulness meditation can help with psoriasis, so if my skin were to also be helped as a by-product that's a bonus.

I like to describe mindful meditation as giving your body a short rest from your busy mind and allowing you to focus on the present moment without judgement. Like most people, my mind darts about from one thought to the next, and I pay little attention to it, allowing my thoughts to come and go. Most of the time, I enjoy my busy mind; I daydream, plan my future, remember my past. It does have downsides though.

If you're thinking about something other than what you're doing at that precise moment in time, you can miss out on the joy of that moment. If I'm walking my dog on the beach but in my head running through all the tasks I need to do at work the following day, I haven't enjoyed the walk, heard the waves crashing, smelt the salty sea air, laughed at my dog as she chases seagulls or noticed our foot and paw prints side by side in the wet sand.

If while I'm walking my dog, I'm replaying a difficult meeting in my mind, my body will react as if that is happening at that exact moment. When I'm worrying about things that happened in the past or may happen in the future, my brain still sends signals to my body to fight or flee the threat. I'll still get a surge of stress hormones, and my heart will pound in my chest, even though I'm safe at that moment in time.

When I practise mindfulness, I don't do anything complex except focus on the here and now. I do it without judgement so I don't tell myself this is a great moment or this isn't as good as I expected, I just notice what's going on around me. Lots of people find it helpful to start by focusing on their breath, but I always find it best to draw my attention to the chair I'm sitting on or the floor beneath my feet. I notice the chair supporting my weight. I notice the material, is it hard or soft? I notice the temperature of the chair. Is it warm or cold? How does the ground feel beneath my feet? Once I've anchored myself to my chair or the ground, I pay attention to my surroundings. What can I hear? What can I smell? What can I see? While I'm doing this, my mind wanders, as our minds have a tendency to do. I just notice that and I refocus on the here and now. This only takes me a couple of minutes, but I try to do it at several points throughout the day, often after parking my car at work and before I start my day, sometimes between appointments and sometimes at the end of the day before I leave work for home.

If you're someone who experiences a lot of stressful and anxiety-provoking thoughts and worries, practising mindfulness will help you take a break from the impact of the stress on your body. It will help you to appreciate the times you are free of stress.

You can download one of many excellent mindfulness apps recommended in the resources section at the end of the book, and these will help you to learn the skills. I also like to encourage people to build mindfulness into their day-to-day lives. How many times have you gone to pick up your mug of tea only to find it empty and you don't remember drinking it? That autopilot mode happens to us all, and it's a sign that you were mind 'full' instead of being present. So instead, if you're having a break with a coffee and a slice of cake, make sure you notice the colours and the textures. Lift the cake to your nose and sniff it. Notice the sensations in your mouth before you take a bite. Savour the flavours on your tongue. And every time your mind wanders away, bring it back to focusing on what you're eating and drinking.

Or, you could take a mindful shower. Instead of dashing in and out, listen to the fall of the water. Feel the water hit your skin. Notice the temperature. Smell the products you're using and take the time in the shower to really appreciate it.

Try this

Take a mindful moment while the kettle boils

Here is a simple mindful exercise you can do while waiting for the kettle to boil:

Put the kettle on and then focus all your attention on your breathing. There's no need to slow down your breathing, just leave your eyes open and breathe as you normally would. Count at the end of each outbreath.

Your mind will wander, that's normal, so be ready to notice that and bring your attention back to your breath.

Feel the sensations of each breath as it flows into and out of your body. Notice the sensations in your nose, your rib cage, your chest. Notice the temperature of the air as you breathe in and then again when you breathe out. Follow each breath as if it were a wave flowing in and out of your body.

If your thoughts drift away, don't worry. Simply notice that it's happened and come back to focus on your breath. In and out. In and out.

Continue this until the kettle comes to a boil.

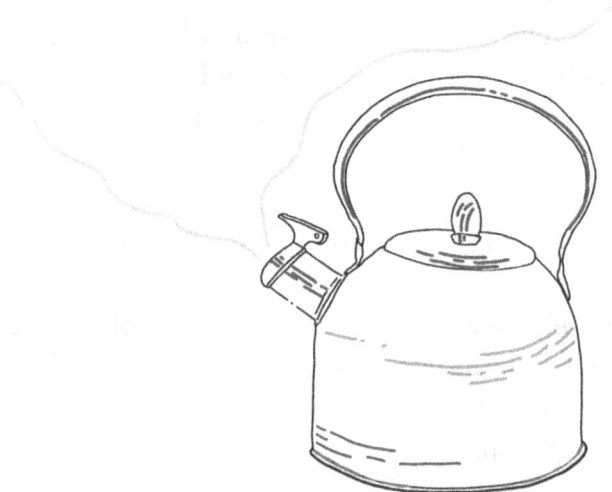

Dennis Potter, the television playwright famous for his sharp writing and psoriasis, taught me the importance of focusing on the present moment back in the 1980s. Growing up in a time without the internet or social media, the only people I met with psoriasis were through a support group, and as they were mainly older women, I didn't really identify with anyone. As a young teenager, Dennis Potter was the only famous person I knew with psoriasis, and he became my role model. When his play *The Singing Detective* was aired on television in 1986, I was both horrified and validated to see psoriasis portrayed on the screen. Potter struggled with both psoriasis and psoriatic arthritis throughout his life. By 1994, he had been diagnosed with terminal cancer. I watched his final interview with Melvyn Bragg, where he talked about the wonder of living in the present moment now that he knew his time was limited. To me, this quote has always impressed upon me the importance of being in the moment, really seeing the world and the people around you. To think that being mindful may also help your physical and emotional well-being is like the cherry on the cake.

> *At this season, the blossom is out in full now ... and instead of saying 'Oh that's nice blossom' ... I see it is the whitest, frothiest, blossomest blossom that there ever could be, and I can see it. The nowness of everything is absolutely wondrous, and if people could see that, you know. There's no way of telling you; you have to experience it, but the glory of it, if you like, the comfort of it, the reassurance. ... The fact is, if you see the present tense, boy do you see it! And boy can you celebrate it. (Potter, 1994)*

Summary

- Lots of people with psoriasis believe stress causes their condition to flare up.
- The evidence to link stress with the onset of psoriasis or the worsening of symptoms is weak.
- Many people feel very stressed by their psoriasis.

- As stress is a normal human emotion, it would be impossible to eliminate from your life.
- Nonetheless, stress feels unpleasant and can have a physiological impact on your body as well as your emotional well-being.
- Psychological strategies can help you manage stress and anxiety.
- Learning to recognise your stress reactions and manage stress in your life may help you feel better, and evidence suggests it may even help improve your psoriasis.

Top tips

- If you feel your stress levels are too high, there are some strategies such as mindfulness that can help.
- Fit mindfulness into your daily routine.
- You can practise mindfulness at any time like in the shower or while the kettle boils.
- The techniques described in Chapters 11 and 12 are also useful for managing stress and anxiety.

4 Psoriasis and shame

I had my hair cut today. If, like me, you have psoriasis on your scalp, you'll understand the stress associated with what most people would consider an ordinary, everyday activity.

I can't face sitting in a busy salon with a dark towel over my shoulders. No matter how good the haircut, the embarrassment would be too much for me to cope with. When I have my hair cut, flakes of skin fall on my shoulders and back, and then onto the floor, where they stand out against the offcuts of my dark hair. There's very little I can do about it. I treat my scalp with ointments prescribed by my doctor, and I wash my hair with a coal tar shampoo. I don't use any styling products at all. Even after phototherapy has successfully cleared the skin on my body, the psoriasis on my scalp remains. Before a hair appointment, I brush as many of the flakes out of my hair as I can, but it's as if my scalp reproduces them just as fast as I remove them. I've always felt embarrassed about having what looks like a devastating case of dandruff.

There is no hiding in a hairdressing salon. I have no control over how busy it is, where I will be seated or who is watching my humiliation. I imagine what other customers are thinking about me: 'Yuck look at her dandruff!', 'Doesn't she know she has dandruff?', 'Why doesn't she do something about it?'. And there is no escape from my shame as I sit scrutinising my reflection in the salon mirror.

In recent years, instead of having to go to a salon, I have found a kind and understanding hairdresser who cuts my hair in the back room of her house. It's just the two of us and I've known her for some time, but even so, I still cringe at the flakes that flurry from my scalp.

Feeling shame

John Updike, the American author, captured the feeling of shame he also felt about his psoriasis:

> *Nov. 1. The doctor whistles when I take off my clothes. 'Quite a case'. ... As I drag my clothes on, a shower of silver falls to the floor. He calls it, professionally, 'scale'. I call it, inwardly, filth.*

Vladimir Nabokov, another writer with psoriasis, also described his feelings of shame and humiliation *'about my bloody underwear, blotchy mug and the scales pouring down on the carpet'*.

Shame is a powerful emotion. It's not exclusive to those of us with psoriasis; most of us feel shame at one time or another. Alongside guilt and embarrassment, shame is described as a moral emotion. It's learnt in childhood following the development of self-awareness and it's thought to promote social hierarchies and prosocial behaviour, encouraging people to behave and act in a way that fits with their culture and societal norms.

Feelings of shame arise from the belief of defectiveness in comparison to others. It's associated with a fear of being judged negatively by others, resulting in low self-worth and humiliation. When people feel shame, it's usually because they believe they have done something, been seen or behaved in a way that is wrong or outside what is desirable. Even when an action hasn't been witnessed, imagined judgement can cause intense feelings of shame and a fear of exposure.

Unlike the other moral emotions such as guilt, where the negative feelings are strongly linked to an action or behaviour (e.g. 'I did something bad'), shame is linked to negative evaluations of the self ('I am a bad person'). When feeling guilty, we focus on the feelings of others, but when feeling ashamed, we focus on ourselves. Our shame supposedly tells us something about the kind of people we are.

With psoriasis, people can feel intense shame because of the way they look and the fear that others will think they're unattractive, disgusting and contagious. The feelings of shame might be linked to entrenched thoughts about the self like 'I'm disgusting' or 'I'm unattractive'.

For those with psoriatic arthritis, shame can arise from not being able to do things they used to or that others would consider simple tasks, like tying up shoelaces or buttoning up a shirt. Not being able to achieve previously desired goals or no longer being able to fulfil valued roles, like working full-time, can cause feelings of shame, just as having to ask for help does.

Societal beliefs about physical perfection

We live in a society where physical perfection is prized and there are strongly held beliefs about what desirable skin should look like: smooth, glowing, unblemished, unlined. These beliefs are promoted in magazines and films and across social media with countless images of people with poreless, flawless skin. We look in the mirror and compare ourselves against filtered and airbrushed photographs of professionally made-up and lit models, setting ourselves unachievable standards.

Those of us with skin conditions also contend with a commonly held misconception that flawless skin equates to healthy skin, and that it is an indication of good internal health. The assumption is that someone with glowing skin is doing all the right things (eating a healthy, nutritious diet, drinking lots of water, getting their eight hours of quality sleep a night, meditating regularly, using the best skin care products); while the person with skin imperfections is doing some, if not all, of these things wrong.

Disgust

Alongside the misconceptions of what healthy skin looks like, people with psoriasis also must contend with the way humans instinctively react with disgust to signs of potentially contagious disease. Disgust is an innate emotion designed to protect an individual from disease, and humans are instinctively disgusted by something that looks like it might be harmful. In the case of skin disease, the feeling of disgust is triggered by visible symptoms, and it leads the disgusted person to keep their distance and hence avoid catching it. Feelings of disgust are more strongly aroused when the person with symptoms is a stranger.

One research study (Pearl et al., 2019) showed photographs of psoriasis to around 400 people, including 187 medical students, some of whom were unfamiliar with psoriasis. Around 40% said they wouldn't shake hands with someone who looked like that, while a third said they wouldn't want someone with psoriasis in their homes. Medical students and people who were familiar with psoriasis or knew someone with psoriasis were far less likely to stigmatise it and reported more compassion and less blame. This suggests that when people know what psoriasis is, and they know it's not contagious, then they are more accepting.

This means that when you have psoriasis, you are dealing with two powerful forces: first, the societal pressures to have flawless skin and be able-bodied; and second, the reactions of those who don't know anything about psoriasis or who believe myths like it's contagious.

We internalise feelings of shame because we not only imagine how people would react to seeing our skin or disability but also because many of us have had real-life experiences of people reacting negatively. The vast majority of participants in one study had experienced people treating them as though they were contagious (Gupta & Gupta, 1995). More than 90% of the sample had experienced strangers making rude or insensitive comments about their psoriasis at some point in their life, while around a quarter had experienced negative comments about their appearance in the month prior to the study. For me, even when comments are intended to be sympathetic and not expressions of disgust, the usual ones being 'ouch, that looks sore' or 'oh poor you', I still experience shame at having skin that others perceive to look painful and that arouses pity.

There have been a few occasions when people have reacted to seeing my skin with quite obvious disgust; while that hasn't happened very often, it's a very painful and upsetting experience.

As a teenager, I had one such incident on a night out with my friends at our local village pub. As the weather was warm, I wore a skirt. I was nervous about exposing the plaques on my legs, but for several weeks I'd had to wear a skirt and ankle socks as part of my school uniform, and while this had been distressing at first, I had become somewhat numbed to my feelings of shame at school.

On this particular night, I stood with my friends in the main bar, and we were chatting and enjoying ourselves. There was a table of young men behind us, and I could hear them laughing and at the same time making noises and expressions of disgust. At this point, I didn't know they were referring to me until one of them said, 'she looks diseased'. Then another of the group reached out and touched my leg, actually pushed his finger into a plaque on my leg and as he did yelled out in mock horror much to the amusement of his friends. I stood there frozen to the spot. My friends moved around me protectively and with my heart pounding in my chest and tears filling my eyes, I spent the rest of the evening in silence and counted down the minutes until my lift home arrived and I could escape. It's left me with an internal scar that has been hard to heal. Profound experiences in childhood like this one shape our deeply held core beliefs about ourselves, other people and the world around us. These core beliefs play an essential role in the development and maintenance of psychological difficulties (Padesky, 1994). As an adult, I can see that the shame of that incident isn't my burden to carry but I've carried it all the same.

If you've had similar experiences, you'll know it's not easy to erase the memories and the impact they have on how you feel about yourself. This incident happened at a particularly sensitive time in my life. Adolescents are generally more prone to feelings of shame than at other times in their lives. For someone like me who had very severe and poorly treated psoriasis throughout my teenage years, alongside having to conform to rules like participating in swimming lessons and wearing a navy-blue school uniform, which meant I couldn't always hide, it was virtually impossible to avoid intense feelings of shame on a regular basis.

Concealment and avoidance

I've continued to battle with feelings of shame for most of my life. It leads me to hide my skin and go to extreme lengths to make sure my true appearance is not revealed. I've spent a lifetime avoiding activities and events, and planning outfits to hide my skin and the flakes and scales that fall from my body and scalp.

I'm not alone in feeling ashamed about the appearance of my skin and the flakes that constantly scatter around me. A study of over 900 people with psoriasis found that shame was one of the most common emotions experienced (Sampogna et al., 2012). Participants didn't seem to get used to having psoriasis: the longer they'd had it, the more shame they reported. Shame also had a serious impact on the lives of people in this study; higher levels were associated with a lower level of educational attainment and difficulties in daily activities.

It's easy to see how that happens. When we feel ashamed, we conceal our skin and avoid certain situations, and that limits our opportunities in life. Shame doesn't just stop us from going swimming or wearing T-shirts on hot days, it also stops us from applying for jobs, pursuing our goals and fulfilling our potential.

Compass of shame

Psoriasis, and the shame we feel because of it, has a huge impact on our most important relationship: our relationship with ourselves. Attempts to deal with shame can lead to emotional and social problems.

The compass of shame model (Nathanson, 1992) explains how, by attempting to cope with feelings of shame, people can end up feeling depressed or withdrawn. This model describes the four ways in which people deal with the negative feelings of shame (Figure 4.1).

i. attacking self by becoming self-critical, leading to depression and low self-worth;
ii. attacking others, leading to anger and aggression;
iii. hiding from self by distracting oneself, leading to addiction problems and thrill-seeking or risky behaviour;
iv. hiding from others, leading to withdrawal, social isolation and loneliness.

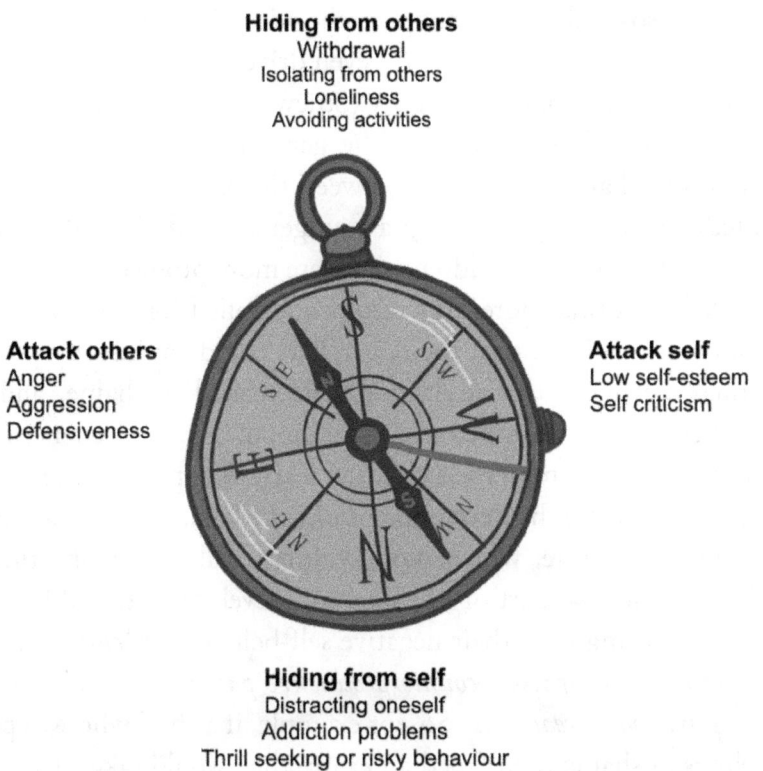

FIGURE 4.1 The psoriasis compass of shame. Source: Adapted from Nathanson, 1992

People may engage in a combination of these coping responses. The self-criticism, low self-esteem and social withdrawal that arise due to attempts to manage feelings of shame can make us vulnerable to a range of mental health problems.

There's a strong link between shame and depression, and between shame and anxiety, particularly social anxiety. One of the axes of the Compass of Shame model suggests that people may respond to shame with anger and aggressive behaviour, and there's evidence this is the case. In particular, people who have a tendency towards feeling shame are quicker to lose their temper in response to criticism, rather than having an angry temperament per se (Hejdenberg & Andrews, 2011). It's proposed that this is a defensive response to humiliation.

There's also evidence to support the idea that in order to avoid uncomfortable feelings, shame can even drive us to self-medicate with alcohol, drugs and food. One study (Stuewig et al., 2015) interviewed 380 American schoolchildren in the general population and found that levels of shame in children between the ages of 10 and 12 years old predicted drinking alcohol at a younger age and illegal drug use as a young adult, with the children who were more prone to shame being more likely to drink more. The results controlled for risky behaviour in childhood, which meant the researchers could confidently propose that these behaviours in adulthood were related to shame, and not simply behaviours continued from childhood. The researchers suggest that the way the shame-prone children learn to cope with these negative feelings leads to the development of risky behaviours. In addition, experiences of failure, which most children will feel at one time or another as a normal part of learning and development, will be taken as evidence fitting with their negative self-beliefs thus *'culminating in an escalating cycle of risky, counterproductive patterns of behaviour and maladaptive shame reactions'*. So, for example, if a child who was prone to feelings of shame then failed an exam, they would take that as evidence of their poor academic ability (ignoring the fact that the whole class failed), thus leading to more feelings of shame. In order to cope with these uncomfortable feelings, they are more likely to engage in risky behaviour like skipping school, smoking and drinking.

Engaging in behaviours like drug use and overeating is also known to cause feelings of shame, and if a disposition towards shame increases the likelihood of these behaviours, then it's easy to see how this can become a negative spiral of shame leading to risky behaviour, and risky behaviour leading to increased feelings of shame.

Impact of shame on physical health

Besides affecting our mental health, feelings of shame can also affect our physical health. Shame causes our bodies to release various stress hormones, including cortisol and pro-inflammatory cytokines (Dolezal & Lyons, 2017).

Over a long period of time, this physiological consequence of shame will cause wear and tear on the body and increase the likelihood of health conditions such as weight gain, heart disease and hardening of the arteries.

Shame and severity of psoriasis

Although one might predict that feelings of shame are related to the severity of psoriasis, with feelings of shame increasing in intensity alongside more severe psoriasis, that doesn't seem to be the case. In one study (Homayoon et al., 2020), the researchers looked at how shame about the skin related to several factors, including an expert-measured disease severity index, the Psoriasis Area and Severity Index (PASI). They found that expert ratings of severity were not associated with the level of shame. This means that you can't predict how much shame a person will be feeling from how severe their psoriasis is. People with less severe psoriasis might be just as vulnerable to feelings of shame. There is evidence that suggests the longer you've had psoriasis, the more shame you are likely to feel (Aberer et al., 2020).

Understanding shame

Overall, it's clear that shame is a destructive and unhelpful emotion. It impacts mental health, physical health and lifestyle choices. In people with psoriasis, it's commonly experienced regardless of the severity of the condition. Feelings of shame can remain even after treatment and even when your skin is clear. Over time, you're likely to feel more shame about your psoriasis.

That all makes for a depressing read, but the good news is that there are things you can do about it. Understanding why shame arises and the consequences of feeling shame is important. By reading this chapter, you will have already raised your awareness of your own feelings of shame instead of them being a hidden but powerful force in driving your behaviour as well as your feelings about yourself.

Acknowledge and accept shame

So, what can you do about your feelings of shame? The most important thing you can do is acknowledge your feelings and accept that they're a normal human reaction to having psoriasis. I know that shame is a universal emotion. I also know that growing up with psoriasis led me to develop a critical and judgemental voice about my appearance. It tells me my skin looks awful, that people would be shocked and disgusted if they see it, that people wouldn't want to be around me if they could see it. I know these thoughts stem from my feelings of shame.

Try and notice what your voice is saying to you. When you catch a glimpse of your reflection after a shower, does it immediately and automatically tell you how disgusting you are? We tell ourselves these things so often that we don't ever stop to question how accurate or helpful our internal voice is being. We just accept them. Instead, when you notice self-critical thoughts like this, ask yourself whether you'd say the same thing in the same tone of voice to a loved one or a friend with psoriasis. It's probable that you wouldn't say that to someone you loved. You'd know it wouldn't help them and would only make them feel bad about themselves, so why turn it on yourself?

The importance of empathy

Instead, it can help to work on developing your self-compassion. You can read about compassion-focused therapy in Chapter 12. Instead of self-criticism, practise treating yourself with kindness, forgiveness and compassion.

Brené Brown is a sociologist who has spent many years researching shame. In a powerful TED talk 'Listening to Shame', she said:

> *Empathy's the antidote to shame. If you put shame in a Petri dish, it needs three things to grow exponentially: secrecy, silence and judgement. If you put the same amount in a Petri dish and douse it with empathy, it can't survive. The two most powerful words when we're in struggle: me too.*

You need to develop empathy for yourself and it's also important to connect with others who have psoriasis. It helps me enormously to see photographs of people who aren't hiding their psoriasis. I look with interest to see how mine differs from theirs, I admire their confidence, I look at other things aside from their skin like their background and their outfit, I absolutely do not feel disgusted. Not even a tiny bit. This helps me to correct my own core belief that my psoriasis looks disgusting. If I don't think their skin looks disgusting, then that means psoriasis isn't disgusting, so how can it be possible that mine is?

The Get Your Skin Out campaign encourages people to share images of their psoriasis on social media. While you might not choose to take part, it can help to see other people, to see they don't feel shame, which can make you realise their skin is not something to be ashamed of. This might help you to be braver about leaving the house in a T-shirt and shorts.

The actress Cara Delevingne went to the Met Gala 2022 in an outfit that not only didn't hide her psoriasis, but instead drew attention to it. Her body, from the waist up, was either wrapped or painted in gold, except for her tattoos and her psoriasis. She used her very public platform to show the world that she doesn't need to cover her psoriasis and she's proud of who she is. Her acceptance of her skin was a powerful reminder to me that you don't need to hide psoriasis and you don't need to feel ashamed.

I think there's more awareness of psoriasis now than there was when I was a child. But even so, there's still work to be done in increasing understanding of psoriasis in the general population. We know that when people are familiar with psoriasis, they are less likely to respond to it in a negative way, so raising awareness helps to reduce stigma. Organisations like the Psoriasis Association and the National Psoriasis Foundation do a lot of good work in promoting awareness and helping to break myths that psoriasis is contagious or is the result of poor hygiene. Social media is another great way to build awareness. Many people post photographs of themselves on Instagram using hashtags like #psoriasiswarrior. Psoriasis awareness month in August is also a good time to share information and reduce stigma.

It's easy to respond with feelings of shame if someone says something insensitive to you. I'm not alone in experiencing discrimination and stigmatisation because of my skin. Having a prepared response ready to use in such situations will mean that you feel calmer and less stressed. This will mean you're less likely to feel upset by the comments and less likely to react in such a negative, unhelpful manner. See Chapter 5 for a full explanation of how to do this. Besides having your response ready, when faced with discrimination or stigma, remind yourself that their reaction is ignorance and you have an autoimmune disease which is not your fault.

Support of others

Getting support from your family and friends can also help, so don't hide your feelings away from them. A case study reported in the journal of *Clinical and Experimental Dermatology* showed that family therapy might not only help people with psoriasis to manage feelings of shame but may also help to clear the skin (Shah & Bewley, 2014). In this case, the patient was a 46-year-old woman who described herself as wearing her psoriasis as 'a badge of shame'. She had tried many treatments prior to the family therapy including biologics, systemic treatments which target specific parts of the immune system, and none had been successful. The psychological intervention consisted of 10 sessions of family therapy; 50-minute sessions with the woman and her husband and one session with her sisters. Over seven months, the therapy focused on family dynamics as well as their beliefs and assumptions about psoriasis. The therapy also involved exploring the patient's core beliefs developed in childhood which were contributing to low self-esteem. At the end of therapy, the patient reported feeling more confident with better self-esteem and her psoriasis had also cleared. While the outcome of a case study can't be generalised, it does raise the importance of support from others in addressing shame.

Our instinct is to hide our shame and not tell others about the way we're feeling, so it will take courage to open up. Brown (Brown, 2006) argues that 'speaking your shame' can help in the development of shame resilience and will help you get some perspective on it.

Empathic relationships appear to be key. There's evidence (Brown, 2006) that stronger, more meaningful relationships allow us to address our feelings of shame. Having someone who totally understands and has walked in your shoes is crucial in developing shame resilience. This means that connecting with other people with psoriasis can be a powerful way to reduce feelings of shame. There are many ways to connect with people with psoriasis (including local groups and online support communities; see the information at the end of the book regarding the Psoriasis Association support forums). I would encourage you to explore your options for connection and reach out and start a conversation. As Brown (Brown, 2021) tells us, 'Shame needs you to believe that you're alone. Empathy is a hostile environment for shame'.

Summary

- People with psoriasis commonly report feelings of shame.
- Shame is associated with the fear of being judged negatively by others.
- Shame can impact physical and mental health.
- Shame can make you hide your skin and withdraw.
- Your shame is not helping you.
- There are things you can do to help reduce your feelings of shame, and empathy is a powerful tool.

Top tips

- Treat yourself with the same kindness and compassion you would use for others.
- Talk about your feelings of shame with your friends and family.
- Connect with other people with psoriasis.

5 Dealing with unwanted attention and others' reactions

Since developing psoriasis, I have had to deal with other people asking questions and commenting on my skin. When I tell my friends about this, they often express surprise that others would be rude enough to draw attention to my psoriasis, but I'm guessing the people who comment usually don't perceive their attention as rude. Most of the time, it's just thoughtlessness or genuine curiosity, and they're often people who aren't very good at putting themselves in someone else's shoes.

There are other times though when people are unkind and that's harder to deal with. Unwanted attention, whether thoughtless or unkind, happens often when your psoriasis is visible. Unless you hide away from the world, learning how to deal with unwanted attention is an important part of learning to cope with psoriasis.

Unwanted attention

People pointing at my skin or asking questions has occurred frequently throughout my life. As a child, people directed their questions and opinions to my Mum rather than me, and I had to stand awkwardly and listen to my health being discussed. When I was backpacking across Asia in my twenties, it was almost impossible to go a day, even in the remotest of places, without someone telling me about the virtues of a well-known skin balm and how it would cure my 'skin problem'.

I still cringe about an incident when I was a trainee clinical psychologist at the Institute of Psychiatry. There I was, a junior psychologist in the canteen surrounded by the great and the good of the mental health world, when a senior tutor smiled knowingly at me and said he knew what I'd been up to the previous night. I had no idea what he was talking about and continued to feel puzzled and confused by his nods and winks, until he eventually pointed at a plaque on my neck describing it as my 'love bite'. I was absolutely mortified and wondered how many of my colleagues and tutors had also noticed it and thought I was unashamedly displaying my love life at work. Was this the only person to say what everyone else had been thinking about me? When I explained to him it was psoriasis, he was mortified at his mistake and now I had to manage both of our feelings of discomfort. I was also left with the dilemma of how to hide the plaque on my neck. Even covering it up with makeup would look like I was trying to hide something. I felt like I needed to wear a sign around my neck explaining that I had psoriasis and not a love bite.

Learning to deal with unwanted attention

Even as a senior clinical psychologist, I've had unwanted attention. One day, I decided to wear a dress to work as the weather was warm and the ward was even warmer. Before I left for work, I asked my family whether the plaques on my legs looked okay and they reassured me they did. That morning started with a busy ward round where a team of specialists followed a consultant around the ward from bedside to bedside, discussing each patient's management plan. This particular morning, I happened to be on the ward but not part of the ward round. As I made my way past my colleagues, one of them looked up and shouted, 'What's happened to your legs, Catherine? Has something been biting you?' and everyone, staff and patients included, turned and craned their necks to get a good look. But by this time, I had learnt a strategy for managing unwanted attention, which meant I dealt with it swiftly and confidently, and I didn't feel ashamed, stressed or embarrassed.

I learnt this strategy when I was working with the cleft lip and palate service in Guy's Hospital in London. Like those of us with psoriasis, children and adults with a cleft lip and/or palate have to deal with questions, comments and unwanted attention. When the visible difference is on someone's face, it's much harder to hide, so it was crucial that the children I was working with learnt how to manage this attention. We can't control the behaviour of other people and we can't stop them from drawing attention to our differences. We can only control our own behaviour and the way we react and feel about it. So, as a psychologist working in a cleft service, my goal was to teach strategies to help lessen the negative impact of other people's behaviour.

Explain-reassure-distract

I leaned heavily on the advice of the excellent charity Changing Faces and not only taught my patients the Explain-Reassure-Distract method to deal with questions and comments but internalised the approach at the same time. This method is simple but effective.

Try this

In response to a question like 'What's wrong with your skin?' you would first give an explanation:

Explain: 'I have psoriasis'.

It needn't be any longer or more in depth than that, though if you want to, you could add something like, 'It's a common autoimmune condition'. You might want to take the opportunity to educate the person about psoriasis. Don't be afraid to give them a ten-minute lecture on the biopsychosocial model of psoriasis if you want to. After all, they asked.

The next thing you need to do is add some reassurance like:

Reassure: 'It's not catching. Don't let it bother you'. Or 'I know it looks sore but I'm getting treatment'.

> The final thing you need to do is distract attention away from your psoriasis, like:
>
> **Distract**: 'Have you been here before?' or 'Did you see the football last night?'
>
> This is the part people think will be most difficult, that is until they've tried it. It's remarkably easy to take control of a conversation and steer it in any direction you choose. Most people are easily and willingly distracted and love nothing better than to talk about themselves and their opinions. Once you've tried it a few times, you start to feel more confident about taking charge, directing the conversation elsewhere, and limiting its potential to cause you upset.

With the incident on the ward, I could have become upset by the question and everyone's attention on my legs and a whole day ahead with them on display. Instead, that particular morning, I took a deep breath and said, 'It's psoriasis (Explain). It doesn't hurt but I really need a sunny holiday to clear it up (Reassure). Can I catch you later to talk about the meeting this afternoon? (Distract)'. Instead of spending the rest of my day distressed, I felt calm and confident and many of my colleagues had smiled and agreed they needed a holiday too. So, there was less discomfort all round and I was able to see that my colleague who asked was not trying to embarrass me or be unkind, which helped protect my feelings of self-worth (Figure 5.1).

Be prepared

I'd recommend having a think about what you would say in such a situation. It really does help to have given it some thought beforehand and feel prepared. Try out different ways of explaining, reassuring and distracting. Choose your own words, and once you have an idea, it's worth trying them out on your family or friends or practising in front of the mirror.

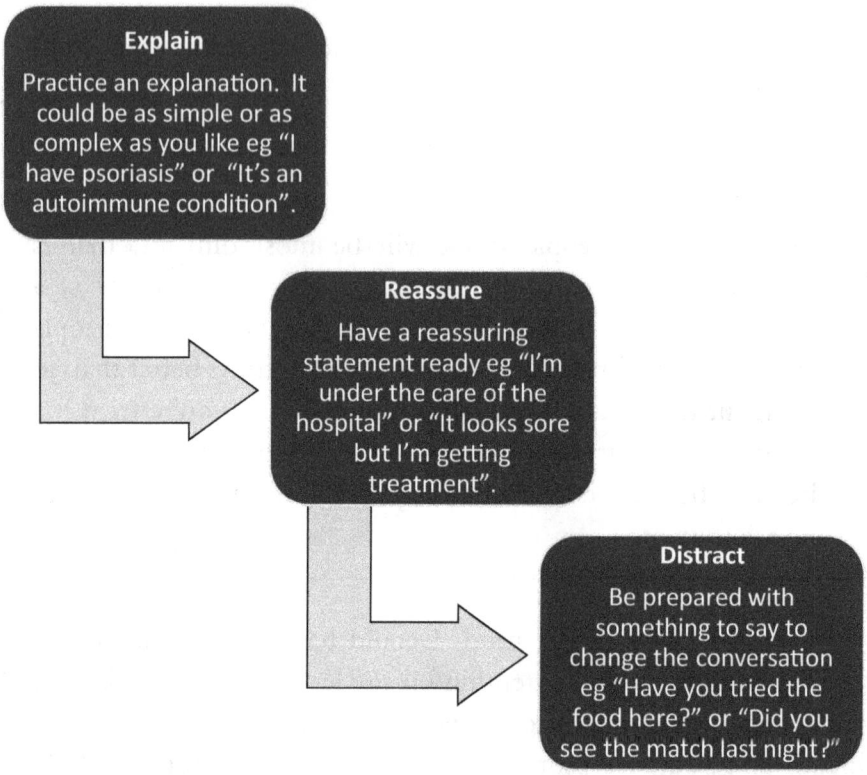

FIGURE 5.1 The psoriasis Explain, Reassure, Distract technique

If you have a child with psoriasis, practise the technique with them so they can use it at school. Instead of getting cross if someone asks you what is wrong with your child, you could take the opportunity to model an 'explain, reassure, distract' response so your child can learn from watching you. Be prepared and then you won't get upset, flustered or angry in the heat of the moment.

Taking control

James Partridge and Adam Pearson are two inspirational men who have written about living with visible differences (Partridge & Pearson, 2008). They suggest that if you have a disfigurement you need to be more socially skilled to help manage the reactions of others. Both

James, who was badly burnt in a car accident, and Adam, who has type 1 neurofibromatosis, a rare genetic condition which causes growths on nerve endings and the skin, have learnt to do this:

James:

> *I experimented with different levels of eye contact, handshake, verbal energy and body language, and found out and eventually mastered the skills to deal with the scared-ness I met – 'scared' being an acronym for staring, curiosity, anguish, recoil, embarrassment and dread. These skills mediated the effect of my outside and boosted my inside too.*

Adam:

> *I discovered too how to control a social situation – just going up to someone who is staring or acting funny and saying 'Hi' is a really good way of breaking the ice and showing your human side.*

Like James and Adam, learning to deal with other people's reactions will take practise and it's a process of trial and error. Some of the young people I worked with in the cleft service were excellent at giving witty and cutting replies to unkind comments that were intended to hurt like 'Remember when I asked for your opinion? Me neither?' or 'Someday you'll go far. I hope you stay there'. That's not for everyone, but if humour is your thing, don't be afraid to use it.

Sometimes you might choose to be assertive, so don't be afraid to walk away from a situation or have a short statement prepared like, 'Please stop staring at me'. This can help you feel in control and get you out of an unpleasant encounter. You may remember in Chapter 4, I wrote about a horrible experience where a group of young men laughed at me in a local pub. This would have been a good time to assert myself. Instead of freezing, I could have walked to a different part of the pub or if I'd felt confident enough, I could have said, 'Please don't make fun of me'. I know my friends would have backed me up.

Other times, you might not want to talk about your psoriasis at all, in which case you can say something like, 'I'd rather not talk about it if you don't mind'. All these responses are perfectly acceptable. The main thing is that you come out of the encounter with your self-esteem intact.

Managing bullying

Sometimes people are downright rude or unkind. Many people with psoriasis report being teased, taunted and bullied because of their psoriasis, especially during adolescence (Magin et al., 2008). Bullying, including teasing, name-calling and taunting, includes verbal and physical aggression, as well as social exclusion or leaving people out. People who have experienced bullying because of their appearance are more likely to feel depressed and anxious and have low self-esteem. Teasing about psoriasis in an Australian study (Magin et al., 2008) was not perceived to be good-natured banter but instead felt negative and hurtful and was often used as a power dynamic to show superiority over someone.

The National Psoriasis Foundation surveyed young people with psoriasis and found that in the previous six months, around half had experienced bullying, including teasing, name-calling and being left out by classmates (Mann, 2013). Most reported feeling anxious about it, and for a quarter of the sample, it affected their academic achievements. Bullying is a significant problem, and with increased use of social media, there's a real risk of cyberbullying too.

Bullying, teasing, taunting, name-calling, whether in person or online, is never acceptable. If you have experienced that, here's some advice from the National Bullying helpline (nationalbullyinghealpline.co.uk):

1. Try to avoid the bully when you're alone.
2. Try not to react to the bully and show you're upset or afraid.
3. If you can, tell the bully to stop.
4. Tell someone you trust and ask for help.
5. Keep a diary of the incidents.
6. If you are being bullied online, delete or block that person. Be wary of giving out your personal details online.

In the spotlight

Most of the time, unwanted attention is 'insensate', that is, it's thoughtless but not intended to upset or hurt. Nonetheless, for me, the experience of unwanted attention has made me anticipate reactions from other people all the time. It's in part linked to a psychological phenomenon known as the spotlight effect.

Most people believe there is more attention on them than there is in reality. It's as if all of us believe we are walking around with a spotlight shining down on us and we are the centre of the world; everyone around is noticing how we look, what we say and how we behave. This makes us acutely self-aware. But here's the thing, if we're all walking around with an imaginary spotlight and focusing on ourselves, and so is everyone else, then who are the people scrutinising everyone else? The truth is they don't exist. We are all living our lives in the glare of our own imagined personal spotlight, whether we have psoriasis or not. This means that most people are more concerned about the way *they look* than the way *you look*. Even if people notice your skin, it won't really matter to them as much as it does to you.

It can come as a shock if someone comments on your skin, and this can strengthen your belief in your own personal spotlight. We need to remind ourselves, that although we remember those incidents clearly, only a tiny proportion of people we have encountered in our lives have stared or commented or asked questions.

The majority of people we have met either didn't notice our skin or didn't care about our skin. Knowing that can dim our spotlight a bit and help us get on with life. It still surprises me when people find out I have psoriasis and they tell me they've never noticed it. In my mind, it's glaringly obvious. But those plaques on my face and body and flakes on my shoulders just aren't as significant to other people.

Putting negative perceptions into perspective

It's also important to be aware that sometimes we incorrectly perceive attention to be negative because of our expectations and previous experiences. A psychology experiment carried out in 1980 took a group of women and made them up with fake scars (Kleck & Strenta, 1985). The women, who thought they were 'disfigured', then had a conversation with a stranger who knew nothing about the experiment. After the conversation, the 'disfigured' women felt stigmatised. They were more aware of the stranger's behaviours like staring and related this to their appearance. They thought the stranger was reacting negatively to the scar and this affected how favourably they rated the stranger.

What the women didn't know was that the experimenters told the women that the fake scar needed to be touched up, but instead had actually removed the scar before the conversation took place. Any negative reaction to the (non-existent) scar was imagined. This study tells us that believing you look different heightens your awareness of other people's behaviour and you are more likely to interpret their behaviour as negatively related to your appearance, whether or not that is actually the case. Because of this, you are more likely to feel uncomfortable around strangers, and this may affect your ability to develop new friendships.

Other approaches

Learning how to handle attention, real or imagined, has helped me to feel more confident about letting people see my psoriasis and that's meant I haven't missed out on things as much as I could have done. Having said that, facing the world, plaques and all, takes a great deal of courage. Like all things, it gets easier with practice, but there may be times when you don't want to show your psoriasis and that's fine too. I've become a master of disguise over the years which gives me confidence about going out. My tips include:

1. Using camouflage make-up. Having a consultation with a specialist in camouflage make-up who matched the make-up to my exact skin tone was absolutely revolutionary for me. It gave me a feeling of control that I'd never felt before, and this helped my confidence in planning future events, feeling safe in the knowledge that if I was to develop a new plaque somewhere visible,

I could hide it if I needed to. The make-up even stays on when swimming. In the UK, you can access a consultation through the Changing Faces charity. The Changing Faces website has lots of advice about how to apply make-up and even recommends high street brands to use if you can't get a consultation.
2. Finding clothes I love in lighter colours with long sleeves helps me feel in control and happy about my appearance. I've found it's no good settling for something when you are under time pressure to buy an outfit. I've learnt to buy clothes that fit my criteria and that I love when I see them.
3. I wear scarves all the time. I feel more confident that I won't have flakes on my back and shoulders if I can regularly shake out a scarf.
4. I found tights or pantyhose made for ice skating are thick enough to hide plaques but still look like flesh-coloured tights. I wore a pair to my sister's wedding and no one noticed the psoriasis on my legs.
5. I have a range of swimming costumes that cover different areas of my body depending on which part I want to hide; rash vests to cover my arms, swimming shorts to hide my thighs, a beautiful burkini which covers my arms and legs (there's a huge range of modesty swimwear available) and wetsuits for colder days. This has meant I can swim in public without fretting about what people are thinking about my skin.
6. Join a psoriasis support group or forum and see what other tips people have for disguising their psoriasis.

The only holiday I've ever had where my first trip down to the pool didn't feel stressful was at the Dead Sea. The resort was full of people with dermatological conditions; at the pool, floating in the Dead Sea, at the hotel restaurant and bar. There was an area set aside on the roof of the hotel specifically for people with psoriasis to sunbathe without clothes. They were single-sex areas and it was perfectly set up with enormous fans, sunbeds and regular deliveries of ice lollies and watermelon to keep us hydrated. I can't tell you how liberating that felt. We bonded across cultures and languages over our psoriasis. I felt absolutely no shame at walking into breakfast in shorts with psoriasis covering my legs. I felt no disgust at seeing other people's psoriasis or other skin conditions, just a huge amount of empathy and comradeship. It was a wonderful learning experience for me.

I would encourage you not to hide away and instead try to deal with unwanted attention, as well as your own ideas about what others might be thinking about you. But don't be hard on yourself if you don't feel confident enough. You may have lived with psoriasis for a long time and have experienced unpleasant reactions from others, and it's understandable that you feel cautious. Sometimes disguising it is just what you need to get through something, and that's okay too.

Summary

- When you have a skin condition like psoriasis, people sometimes stare, comment or ask questions.
- This unwanted attention can feel distressing.
- Preparing yourself for unwanted attention will help you feel more in control and less stressed.
- The Explain-Reassure-Distract method can help you feel in control and turn the attention away from your psoriasis.
- Sometimes the attention is meant to be hurtful. That is never okay.
- You may want to disguise or hide your psoriasis at times, and that's okay too.

Top tips

- Be prepared for unwanted attention with an Explain, Reassure, Distract response.
- Practise and then give it a go.
- Taking control will help you deal with questions, comments and stares.
- Remember that other people's attention is focused on their own spotlight.

6 Living with pain, discomfort and itching

Pain has an element of blank;
It cannot recollect
When it began, or if there were
A day when it was not.

— EMILY DICKINSON

Skin covers the whole surface of our body. It has an important job as both a barrier and an interface between us and our environment. It detects temperature and helps us to regulate according to our surroundings. It protects us from foreign bacteria and viruses, and it's also designed to alert us to sources of danger like sharp implements and extreme heat or cold.

Pain receptors

Skin achieves these vital tasks through a network of tiny sensory receptors found close to the surface. They send signals to our spinal cord and brain about the environment. The most numerous of the receptors in our skin are pain receptors; every square centimetre contains around 200. Together, the receptors alert our nervous system when something isn't right. That way, we know there's a stone in our shoe, if the radiator we're sitting next to is too hot or that we've cut ourselves and need to attend to it.

It's not surprising, then, that many people with psoriasis report experiencing pain. The receptors respond to dry, inflamed and flaky skin by sending messages of pain and discomfort to our brains. If I had a stone in my shoe, receptors would alert me, and I would take off my shoe to shake it out. But with psoriasis, there is no stone to remove, so

I'm left with firing receptors signalling my brain with little chance to alleviate the pain.

My experience of pain from psoriasis varies and can be intermittent. My skin often feels sore, burning hot and stretched, I feel discomfort and I itch. The psoriasis in my ears drives me crazy in a way that someone could only understand if they'd experienced it. Various joints in my fingers, toes and elbows throb like toothache. My joints hurt all the time for short periods, and then there'll be long periods without any joint pain at all. The pain in my nails, particularly my toenails, can be excruciating, especially if I bang my foot accidentally and stub my toes. It's a sharp pain that brings tears to my eyes.

Types of pain associated with psoriasis

People with psoriasis report a range of pain experiences, including

- tight, itchy skin on scalp
- burning sensation
- itching inside ears
- eye inflammation
- painful joints
- swollen fingers and toes
- pitted, thickened, crumbling nails
- heel and foot pain
- sore, dry skin
- tight, red skin
- itchy skin
- cracked and bleeding skin

Estimates of how many people with psoriasis report pain vary widely from 17% in some studies to as much as 83% in other studies (Martin et al., 2015). This is in part due to how we define pain or discomfort. The chronic nature of psoriasis means we also just get used to the way our skin feels and that stops us from being able to tell if we feel discomfort because this is just our normal experience.

One study interviewed people with moderate-to-severe psoriasis and found that skin pain was reported by the majority of those interviewed (Martin et al., 2015). It was described in many ways: 'painful like an open sore', 'a dull pain', 'a sharp stabbing pain', 'an irritating pain' and 'a throbbing and stinging pain'. Besides pain caused by the plaques themselves, a number of people talked about pain caused by unconscious scratching. Those with psoriatic arthritis had the additional issue of painful joints.

In a recent study (Snyder et al., 2022), people with psoriasis reported that their pain was often self-inflicted through picking or scrubbing away flakes to leave raw skin. Scratching was hard to control though, as it provided only temporary relief.

Skin pain and quality of life

There's evidence to suggest that people with skin pain have a worse quality of life, more sleep disturbance and feel more emotional distress (Ljosaa et al., 2012). This is not surprising because being in pain is likely to have an impact on your day and the things you're able to do.

People who experience pain because of their psoriasis are more likely to miss work, they're less productive at work and they are less able to do daily tasks and activities (Lewis-Beck et al., 2013). Because pain associated with psoriasis also affects sleep (Ljosaa et al., 2010), you're more likely to feel tired, unable to cope with daily life and that your overall quality of life is poor.

Pain and mood

Being in pain can also affect your mood. In addition to feeling low, people experiencing pain describe being irritable, impatient and quick to lose their temper. Most studies across a range of different health conditions show that people with ongoing pain are often angry. To illustrate this, I like to think about our capacity to lose our temper as being a firework, and the speed with which we lose it is dependent both on the gunpowder in the body of the firework and the length of a fuse.

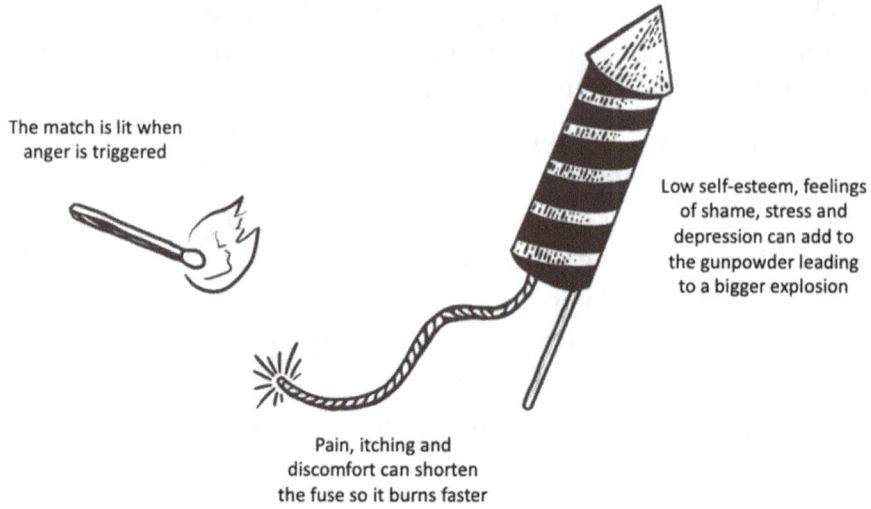

FIGURE 6.1 The psoriasis anger firework

All of us have gunpowder inside our fireworks, and when the fuse is lit, there are things we can do to extinguish the flame and stop the firework from exploding. We might count to five or remove ourselves from the situation, and this can stop us losing our temper. However, your fuse is shortened when you're in pain. If lit, it burns down to the gunpowder quickly, and there's little time between trigger and explosion. Pain gives you a short fuse, and while you can still put it out, it's much harder. We also know that being angry increases the production of stress chemicals like adrenaline and cortisol. Pain-related brain activity increases, which then amplifies the experience of pain. This can become a vicious cycle of pain leading to anger and anger-intensifying pain (Figure 6.1).

Itching

Pruritus or itching is experienced by most people with psoriasis, regardless of how extensive their psoriasis is. Feeling itchy is a normal part of life for me, and my scalp is much itchier than the rest of my body.

I do my best to resist scratching because I know that usually makes things worse, but there are times when I give in to it. After the birth of my third child, the itching was particularly bad. Like all new parents, I was tired, but any time I tried to sleep, I itched intensely all over my body. It was a distressing skin sensation. I could not stop myself from scratching and did so every night for weeks, waking in the mornings covered in blood and sore.

Itching is a form of pain that's hard to deal with. Triggers may include the climate, especially hot or arid conditions, showering or bathing, using perfumed skin products and certain fabrics. Some people have reported that their itchiness is triggered by emotional stress (Taliercio et al., 2021). Itching leads to scratching, which leads to increased flaking, bleeding and open sores, and all that can feel shameful and embarrassing (as we saw in Chapter 4).

There are several theories about why itchiness is such a common symptom. These include complex biological mechanisms, such as the release of neuropeptides from nerve endings in the skin, which results in an itching sensation (Szepietowski & Reich, 2016). Relief from itching seems to be best managed by treating the plaques.

Attentional bias

The experience of itching may also be affected by attentional bias, which is a tendency to focus on certain sensations over others depending on various factors such as our environment or emotions. Even while writing this chapter, I'm more aware of any itchy sensation in my skin, and as a result, I'm feeling more itchy than usual. This doesn't only apply to people with psoriasis. I can remember countless times waiting to collect my children from school, standing at the school gates with the other parents and our children running out to greet us clutching the dreaded, 'there has been an outbreak of nits in your child's class' letter. Parents would instantly start to feel itchy.

Pain management

Reducing itchiness, burning sensation and pain are considered by people with psoriasis to be the most important goals of treatment (Blome et al., 2016), but in all my years of treatment, I don't ever remember being asked about my symptoms of pain or itching. The management of pain in psoriasis has been described as an unmet need since so many people report experiencing it but treatment is rarely offered (Misery et al., 2020).

When I was training, I worked on placement in a pain management team at St Thomas' Hospital in London. The people who attended the residential pain management programme came from all over the UK and had lived with chronic pain, mainly back pain, for a long time, exhausting every treatment option (often including numerous operations and powerful pain medication). The highly successful programme was run by nurses, doctors, physiotherapists, occupational therapists and psychologists.

I was lucky to learn about the management of chronic pain from an internationally renowned team in a centre of clinical and academic excellence. I also learnt a great deal from the people I met who had been struggling with chronic pain for a long time, often many years. As I have always done throughout my career, I pondered the relevance of this for psoriasis. I had never been asked about my experience of pain, yet I had felt it regularly for most of my adult life.

The psychology of pain

You may wonder why a hospital pain team would include health professionals like psychologists. It's not because the pain is considered to be psychological, in someone's head or imagined. The pain is very real but what we know about pain is that certain psychological factors and behaviours can make things worse, and various psychological strategies and techniques can help someone to cope.

If you have ever knocked your elbow or funny bone, you'll know it is certainly not funny and can feel like an intense sharp pain. The science behind it is that your ulnar nerve is squashed into your medial epicondyle bone, resulting in that horrible pain which radiates down your arm and into your fingers.

You might also have noticed that the way you respond to the pain differs according to where you are, who you're with, as well as the way you're feeling.

I could be having a really bad day. I've had some bad news which has made me feel down and worried. And then I knock my elbow. It hurts, it feels like the final straw and I cry to my husband who comforts me. My elbow throbs. Now imagine I'm alone in the house. Do I cry in the same way? Now imagine I'm in a big lecture room and I knock my elbow on the podium just before I'm about to start a keynote presentation. Do I cry then or hop from foot to foot? In one scenario, I cry while I rub my elbow and am comforted. In another scenario, I ignore the pain and start my presentation. It's the same pain, but the way I communicate the pain and the way I respond differs.

In the same way, we don't know if we all experience pain in the same way. People talk about having a high or low pain threshold, but we just don't know if everyone's pain scale is the same. Some people have no trouble coping with dental procedures with no anaesthetic, others need numbing cream before having blood drawn. Pain is subjective; it varies from person to person and for each individual, it varies from time to time, depending on the situation.

'Gate theory' of pain

We know that the pain pathway is complex and much more nuanced than a pain receptor in the skin sending a signal to the brain. People with amputations experience phantom pain, even in the absence of the limb. Psychologists have theorised that the subjective experience of pain is controlled by gateways. Known as the gate theory of pain, this recognises that the brain plays an important role in incorporating a range of information into the pain experience, such as past episodes of pain, levels of anxiety and attention.

The idea behind the gate theory is that the nerves sending pain signals to the spinal cord have to first pass through a series of gates. Sometimes the gates are wide open, at which time the pain signal moves fast to your brain, and sometimes they are only slightly open or closed altogether. When the gates are more closed, the pain signals are less likely to get through. Numerous factors can open the gates like paying attention to the pain, stress and psychological suffering and also lack of activity and overall fitness. The good news is that there are factors under our control that can help to close the gate, like rubbing the spot that hurts or applying heat or mental factors like feeling relaxed or happy. For me, moisturising definitely helps. I think of moisturiser as one of my pain management tools. It doesn't clear or treat my skin, but it softens it enough to stop the pain receptors firing constantly.

It can help to see what's going on when your pain levels are lower. Those might be the very activities that close your gate. You could try the following methods to close the gates, remembering that we're all different and what works for some people might not work for others (Figure 6.2).

Pain-related thinking, like telling yourself you can't cope with the pain, contributes too by opening the gates really wide. Worrying about the pain and paying attention to it also opens the gates. Thoughts like

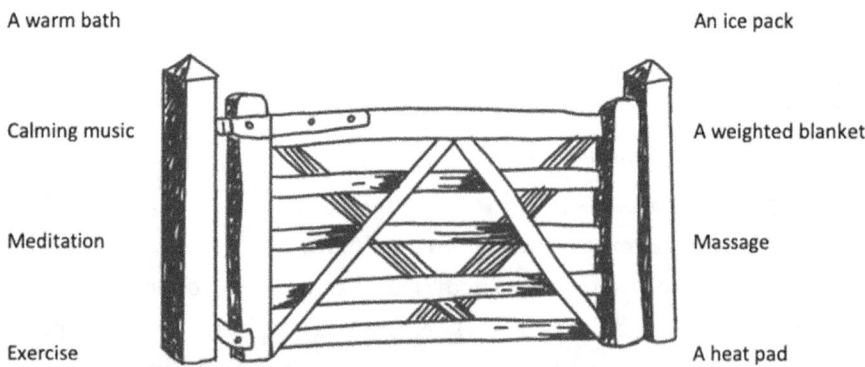

FIGURE 6.2 Methods to close the gate and reduce the psoriasis pain signals

'this is getting worse' might lead you to do less, which not only opens the gate but can lead to decreasing fitness and muscle deconditioning.

It's common to tell yourself that you can't cope and that things will never get better. Negative thoughts about pain are often linked to worries that it will never end and it's insurmountable. Just like the Emily Dickinson poem at the start of this chapter, when you're in pain it's hard to remember when it started or even if there was ever a time without pain. However, these negative thoughts and self-talk influence how we respond to the pain.

Introducing the cognitive defusion technique

People with negative pain-related thoughts are more likely to report being physically disabled, feel less able to overcome the pain, are more fearful of worsening the pain and experience more stress, all of which lead to reduced activity and isolation. It can help to start noticing your negative self-talk about pain and remind yourself that just because you think something, it doesn't make it true. Cognitive defusion is a helpful strategy as it allows you to see thoughts for what they are and not what they say they are. One strategy is to add 'I notice that I'm having the thought that ...' to the beginning of your negative thoughts. For example, 'I notice I'm having the thought that I can't cope with this pain'. This allows you to not get caught up in the feelings and actions that usually follow on from such thinking and can reduce suffering. You can read more about this technique in Chapter 11.

Practical steps to address pain

For me, there are several practical things that close the pain gates. Keeping my skin moisturised always helps, and I have a good routine of applying cream every morning. It's as much a part of my daily life as brushing my teeth. Naturally, my routine slips from time to time, and I always feel more discomfort and pain on the days I miss moisturising.

At times when my skin is particularly sore, it can help to keep ointments chilled in the fridge so they feel extra soothing. It's not practical to moisturise at all times, but I do try to keep small pots of moisturiser with me. I have them in my bag, in my desk at work and in my car.

I also find a bath helpful. If the water is too hot, that can make things worse, so I'm careful to find the right temperature, and I use an emollient in the water. If I'm feeling in pain, I know I find it helpful to turn my attention to something else, like listening to an audiobook or music.

Avoid overdoing things

In conditions like psoriasis, where the pain may be intermittent, you might be inadvertently making the situation worse. It's common for people to try to take advantage of the times when the pain lessens and try to do everything they haven't been able to when the pain is more severe, like walking the dog, cleaning, exercising and keep going until the point of exhaustion. The desire behind this is to make the most of a pain-free moment, but what happens is that by trying to fit everything in, you actually overdo it and trigger a new bout of pain. This then leads to a period of inactivity with the frustration of not being able to do anything. It can lead to a cycle of boom and bust, periods of overdoing, followed by periods of underdoing.

If you suspect you might fall victim to this, you could keep an activity diary and see if a pattern of boom and bust emerges. Try to pace your day. Even if you're feeling great, be aware of the risk of overdoing things and stop before you feel in pain or exhausted.

Pain and sleep

Pain, discomfort and itching can all affect the quantity and quality of sleep you get. Sleep deprivation can make everything feel much worse, and your ability to cope can be diminished. Strategies that help to reduce physical discomfort will help with sleep. Other strategies include:

- Reducing your caffeine intake from late afternoon onwards. That includes tea, green tea, coffee, cola, energy drinks and chocolate. Ideally, give up products containing caffeine altogether. Drink chamomile tea or a milky drink at bedtime instead. Alcohol and nicotine are also stimulants that will disturb your sleep.
- Getting some exercise during the day, something outdoors like walking or cycling so you get some sunlight will be beneficial as natural light is linked to our sleep cycle.
- Getting into a good routine. Go to bed and get up at the same time every day. Get up at your set time, even if you've had a bad night. Try not to nap during the day or sleep late until a good routine has been established.
- Not worrying about not sleeping. If you are lying awake in bed in the wee small hours, don't panic about how tired you will be or how your skin will suffer. Easier said than done, but instead of worrying, use the time to do some mindfulness or another type of meditation. That way you'll be using the time to rest your body even if you aren't asleep.
- Turning your clock to face the wall. Don't be tempted to check what time it is. It doesn't matter and will only cause stress or wake you up. Don't cheat and look at your phone or your watch.
- Making your bedroom relaxing and inviting. My favourite of all is clean sheets, line dried (they smell so good after a day in the sun) and preferably put on the bed by someone else. I may not have a great night's sleep but at least I go to bed happy.

It might be the case that you need less sleep than you used to. Our sleep requirements often reduce as we get older, but we still expect to need the nine hours we had when we were teenagers. It's also quite likely that you're getting more sleep than you realise. Research in sleep laboratories shows that individuals who claim not to sleep get much more than they estimate. See information at the end of the book for helpful sleep resources.

Introducing Acceptance and Commitment Therapy

Acceptance and Commitment Therapy (ACT) has emerged as a helpful psychological therapy for coping with pain. You can read more about ACT in Chapter 11. The basic idea behind ACT is that the suffering associated with pain isn't essential. ACT doesn't try to cure or control the pain, instead it's an alternative to suffering that pain normally brings.

Many ACT therapists use a metaphor that likens living with pain to being in a tug of war battle with a monster. You're on one side of the rope and the monster is on the other, and between is a deep, dark hole. The monster is pulling you towards the hole and you are pulling on the rope with all your might. Everything is focused on the struggle. You stop doing the things you love and paying attention to what's around you and instead you pull and pull to stop yourself being dragged into the hole.

ACT tells us that this is what happens when we struggle with pain. We fight and resist and put everything into the battle, and our lives shrink down to a struggle with pain.

But what if instead we just dropped the rope and walked away from the tug of war? This might feel confusing, as the pain would still be there. But we need to understand that the pain isn't helped by the struggle. Although it can feel like it's stopping us from being dragged into a hole, the struggle is making our lives miserable. Once the struggle has stopped, you can turn your attention to other things that bring your life joy and meaning. This has the added benefit of closing the pain gates. ACT doesn't encourage you to ignore the pain; instead, it teaches you to acknowledge pain and to stop it defining your life and making things worse.

The relationship between psoriasis, pain and suffering is complex. Figure 6.3 might help make it clearer.

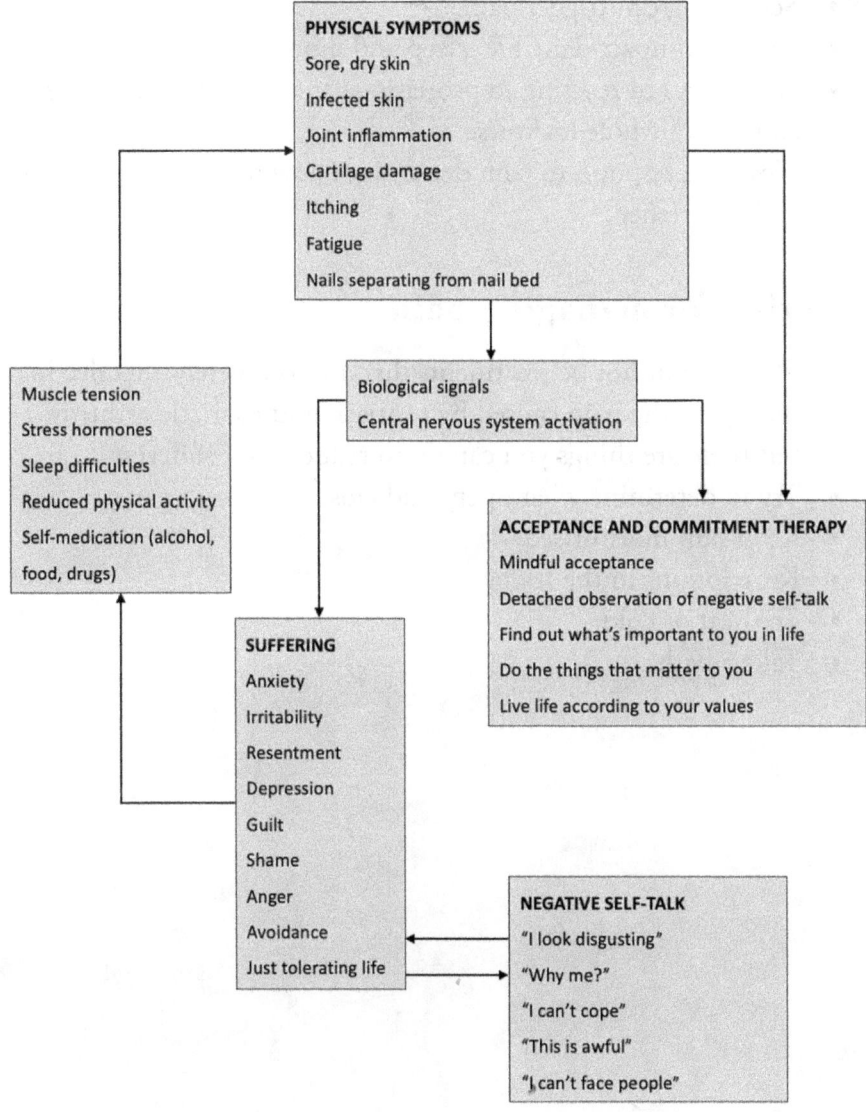

FIGURE 6.3 The complex relationship between psoriasis, pain and suffering

Summary

- Psoriasis is a condition causing physical pain as well as emotional pain.
- Pain can be intense and is felt in the skin as well as in the joints.

- Scratching can trigger pain.
- Pain can impact daily life, sleep and mood.
- Some ways of reacting to psoriasis-related pain can make the situation a whole lot worse.
- How you respond to pain determines how much suffering you will experience.

Top tips for managing pain

- There might not be treatments that are completely effective in managing the pain caused by psoriasis and psoriatic arthritis, but there are things you can do to reduce your suffering.
- Try to determine what opens and closes your pain gates.
- Keep skin moisturised.
- Keep lotions in the fridge.
- Try heat or cold.
- Take a bath.

7 Blame and lifestyle factors

I think about how it's not knowing that torments all of us. At a certain point, we all have to come to terms with the unknown and the unknowable. Sometimes we'll never know why.

— **Lori Gottlieb**, *Maybe You Should Talk to Someone*

The hardship of not knowing

While we know psoriasis is an autoimmune condition and we know there is likely to be a genetic component, no one can ever tell us why we developed psoriasis in the first place. Not knowing why you have psoriasis and why at times it flares up, only to retreat at other times, is extremely difficult to live with. In her memoir, Lori Gottlieb (Gottlieb, 2019) talks about the universal struggle against not knowing, from not knowing what's wrong with your body to not knowing why your boyfriend left you and how this can lead to psychological difficulties.

I've always struggled to accept that my psoriasis is multifactorial and I am constantly searching for answers. Why does it affect my elbows more than other areas on my body? Why do my joints hurt sometimes but not others? Why do the plaques on my scalp suddenly thicken and itch like crazy? The ever-changing nature of the condition means it's only natural that I should ask myself what I'm doing differently to cause these changes. I've spent decades questioning what I'm doing wrong.

Short-lived relief

The other thing for me, as with many people with psoriasis, is that a change in lifestyle or a new treatment often works miraculously the first time I try it, but then never again. Many years ago, my parents bought me some Dead Sea salts. I soaked in the bath and watched as the plaques faded to a pale pink. In the days following, they continued to fade and the scaling stopped. We thought we had the solution, and my parents eagerly ordered a sack of Dead Sea salts straight from the source. But it never worked again. It's a game of cat and mouse, and the small successes and constant fluctuations in symptoms push you to keep trying.

My teen years and twenties were spent in a constant search for a cure. The hope is that you can take back control and do something about it. I would try every miracle cure written about psoriasis in newspapers and magazines. I tried every kind of alternative therapy. Some worked for a short while, but eventually the psoriasis came back.

Falling prey to 'miracle cures'

Once, someone I met at an alternative therapy fair told me she had a cure for psoriasis in the form of a spray imported from the Middle East. I could make an appointment to go to her house to have it applied. She told me it was expensive, very hard to get hold of and so she couldn't give me my own spray to take away, but if I went to her house to have it applied weekly, it would work. Her certainty was very attractive.

At the second appointment, she left the room briefly and I scribbled down the name of the product within the spray canister. This was in the days before mobile phones to take a photograph or the Internet to search it up there and then. Later at home, I called my chemist only to be told that it was a spray barrier lotion available over the counter from any chemist for less cost than a pint of milk. I was crushed with disappointment not only at the alternative therapist's deceit but by the way she'd raised my hopes only to have them dashed so cynically.

Another time, a spray treatment I bought online had rapid and miraculous results, and I spent several weeks clear. Although new patches regularly emerged, they quickly beat a hasty retreat after being sprayed with the 'all natural zinc based' treatment. I bought many cans of it to stock up in case they ran short, and I was delighted with the outcome. Yet, after several weeks, I was starting to suspect things weren't quite as they seemed. I could see my skin thinning, and I was starting to bruise everywhere.

I was not the only person with psoriasis to be wondering about the spray's legitimacy as people online began to raise serious questions. It later emerged that the spray contained a potent, unlisted steroid. That was why it worked so well and why I had one of the worst rebound flare-ups when I stopped using it. That was a very low point, and I decided not to waste any more money on miracle cures.

Self-blame and lifestyle adaptations

I continue to adapt my lifestyle in order to gain some control over my skin. Restricting what I eat and managing the levels of stress I expose myself to have become ingrained habits. I've no doubt this has limited my opportunities in life, but I can't seem to stop feeling guilty when I eat junk food or allow myself to get too stressed.

With psoriasis, perhaps more than other conditions, self-blame seems to be an important factor. The American Academy of Dermatology Association informs us that there are triggers for a flare-up including stress, drinking in excess, smoking, getting tattoos and piercings, and sunburn. Obesity is another factor linked to worsening symptoms. These triggers are all things that could be under our potential control, so it's no wonder we blame ourselves (Figure 7.1). This feeds into the shame we feel, as discussed in Chapter 4.

If you have psoriasis, there's an increased risk of these triggers being a part of your lifestyle as a coping strategy. We learnt in Chapter 4 about a large-scale study in the general population in America (Stuewig et al., 2015) which found that people who were more prone to shame in childhood (between the ages of 10 and 12) were more likely to take risks such as using illegal drugs, drinking alcohol at a younger age and having unprotected sex in adulthood. There's evidence that people with psoriasis drink more than other people (Svanström et al., 2019). The alcohol may worsen symptoms through several mechanisms including increased susceptibility to infection and increased inflammation. People with psoriasis are 60% more likely to die due to alcohol-related illness than the general population (Parisi et al., 2017).

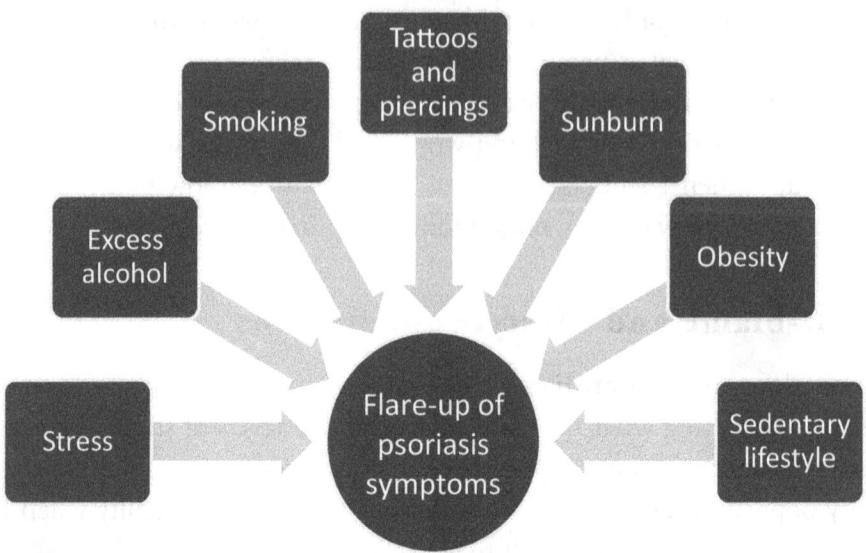

FIGURE 7.1 Potential factors triggering a flare-up

If the stress associated with living with psoriasis increases your risk of drinking and other unhealthy behaviours, and those behaviours then trigger flare-ups in psoriasis, it's easy to see how this could become a vicious cycle. Introducing self-blame into the mix will make things a whole lot worse.

Low self-esteem and self-loathing

It could also follow that blaming oneself for having psoriasis could result in low self-esteem and self-loathing. After all, if it's something I'm doing that's making my skin so bad then surely I deserve it. A study I conducted in collaboration with the dermatology department at King's College Hospital in London found that around 60% of people believed their psoriasis was caused by stress (O'Leary et al., 2004). Those people who believed stress was the main causal factor were significantly more likely to feel depressed and anxious, regardless of the severity of the condition. This suggests that it's not especially psychologically helpful to believe stress is causal, which may link to feelings of self-blame.

Seeking control through diet

For many people with psoriasis, diet seems to be one way to exert some control. We are given messages about the importance of diet for health and in particular healthy skin, so it would seem natural to assume that improvements in what and when we eat and drink could make a difference. A Google search of psoriasis and diet produces countless websites offering advice about what to eat and what to avoid. There are psoriasis cookbooks, recipes with promises of healing and memoirs of people who cleared their psoriasis by 'clean' eating.

I've frequently asked at my clinic appointments about the evidence for diet as a trigger, but I have been told there is little to go on, other than the association of obesity with poorer outcomes. That hasn't stopped me from trying many different diets, from gluten-free to sugar-free to nightshade-free to whole-food plant-based.

I've looked at the scientific research examining the link between diet and psoriasis, and the lack of evidence is due mainly to the difficulty of conducting such studies. Research around the impact of dietary factors on any health condition is notoriously difficult to conduct because people find it hard to follow a restricted diet for an extended period of time. Anyone who knows about the diet industry will tell you that most people have trouble sticking to a prescribed regimen. The experimental group would not only have to be large in number but also motivated, willing and able to follow a restricted diet, without the occasional meal out, holiday or other cheats.

Diet research

Despite the difficulties, there are some interesting studies to note. One study carried out in Croatia (Rucević et al., 2003) gave the experimental group a low-energy diet consisting of nothing but fresh and boiled vegetables, fruit, rice, bread and low-fat dairy for four weeks while they were hospital inpatients. The authors report significant changes in serum lipids (fat-like substances found in blood) as well as improvements in psoriasis which were associated with the reduction in serum lipids. However, we don't know how many of the original 42 people made it to the end of the trial and how many popped out for a sneaky burger on the weekend or kept a bar of emergency chocolate in their hospital locker.

In 2018, the Medical Board of the National Psoriasis Foundation (Ford et al., 2018) looked at the results of 55 studies of diet in psoriasis. The strongest evidence was for the benefits of weight loss for psoriasis in overweight people, but they concluded overall the evidence is just not strong enough to draw any firm links.

There is plenty of anecdotal evidence, much of it emerging from times of war and famine. It has been alleged that in post–World War I Germany, psoriasis all but disappeared from the population. The same was reported in Dutch prisoners of war in World War II concentration camps.

This fits with reported findings from 1970s Russia. The Medical Institute of Dermatology in Moscow (Makeev, 1976) reported on their fasting treatment where people with psoriasis ate and drank nothing except mineral water and vitamins for two weeks and had daily enemas. Not surprisingly, their subjects lost weight, and there was some improvement in the skin which reversed as soon as they started eating normally again.

It would seem that a low-energy diet reduces the severity of psoriasis, though food restriction can lead to other health problems. However, in contrast to this evidence, there are also reports of an increase in the incidence and severity of psoriasis during World War II when food was restricted for many (Lomholt, 1964). The incidence of psoriasis is reportedly low in Eskimo and Danish populations, which has drawn some researchers to link this with their high intake of fish oils and fatty acids. However, Yang and Chi (2019) reviewed several studies looking at the benefits of fish oil supplements in psoriasis and found there was insufficient evidence to recommend it as a treatment.

There is evidence that obesity increases the risk of developing psoriasis (Snekvik et al., 2017) and increases in physical activity can lead to improvements in the condition (Schmitt-Egenolf, 2016). Another longitudinal study of over 35,000 Norwegians found that obesity, particularly around the waistline, is associated with an increased risk of psoriasis. High levels of physical activity decreased the risk regardless of weight (Thomsen et al., 2021). A similar study in the UK found that a decrease in weight over a ten-year period was associated with a reduction in the risk of developing psoriasis (Green et al., 2020).

The risk of orthorexia

Though not a formal diagnosis , orthorexia is a type of eating disorder where there is an obsessive focus on clean or healthy eating. It's associated with restricted eating and the omission of certain types of food groups which are not considered pure, for example eating only raw foods.

Not knowing but suspecting that diet is involved in my psoriasis has led me to be suspicious of food and whether it's harming me. For me, and perhaps for others with psoriasis, there is a risk of developing orthorexia fuelled by the countless websites, books and diets purporting to have the cure through diet. Whenever I read that someone 'cured' their psoriasis by avoiding gluten or tomatoes or by eating 20 blueberries a day, it sows a seed in my mind that is difficult to shift.

I wonder whether I have orthorexia. The strongest of my food-related beliefs is that sugar makes my plaques more inflamed, sore and itchy, so I restrict the amount of sugar I consume. I would never willingly consume sugary drinks and rarely eat confectionary. A slice of cake, ice cream or a chunk of chocolate is always accompanied by a large helping of guilt, which lasts for far longer than the sugary sweetness lingers in my mouth. It's a pleasure–guilt dilemma and guilt always wins out. Yet what if I'm wrong and sugar has no effect at all on my skin? There's a part of me that thinks that even if that's the case, at least I've protected my teeth and heart health. But I know I've missed out on simple pleasures that others take for granted.

This is the constant dilemma of psoriasis. We don't fully understand why we have it or what we need to do to stop new plaques and flare-ups, but we're also told there are triggers like stress, obesity and drinking too much and that exercise and meditation can help. We believe if only we got all these things right, then we'll be in control, and when we fail in our mission, we blame ourselves.

The scientific literature supports this message, telling us that by making lifestyle improvements we could follow a virtuous cycle instead of a vicious cycle (Schmitt-Egenolf, 2016). In the vicious cycle, psoriasis leads to feelings of depression and shame, which then lead to isolation and bad lifestyle choices such as smoking and a sedentary lifestyle, leading to more sudden and severe flare-ups. In contrast, in a virtuous cycle, good lifestyle choices would be made, such as exercise and a healthy diet, and alongside a better awareness of health issues, this would lead to delayed or weaker flares.

Setting up for failure

While I don't deny the benefits of such a healthy lifestyle, I'm 100% confident that I could do all these things and I would still have psoriasis. I also think it's setting me up for failure. Naturally, my life takes unexpected twists and turns. A recent head cold has stopped me from running for the past week, but a broken leg would take me out of action for longer. Changes in my routine and big life events like births, deaths and marriage have large impacts on my diet, my sleep and my stress levels. I'm exposed to stressful events outside my control, factors at work, changes of government, wars and extreme weather. The virtuous cycle is an ideal to strive for but is presented to me as a potential method of treating my psoriasis. The virtuous cycle is a dangerous ideal leading me not on a path to clear skin but to a sense of failure and responsibility (Figure 7.2).

Blame and lifestyle factors

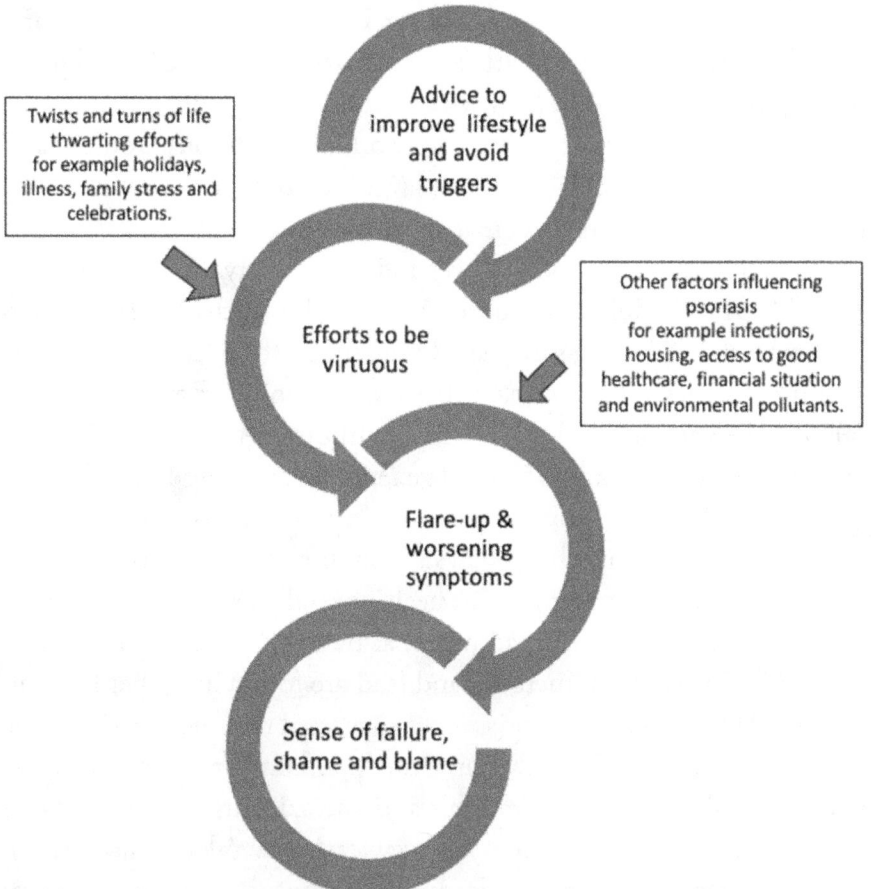

FIGURE 7.2 Challenges of following a virtuous cycle

Other factors at play

Instead of believing that my diet is the biggest factor relating to my skin, and responsible for more than 90% of the redness, flaking and itching, I find it more helpful to widen my thinking and remember all the factors involved.

As far back as 1991, researchers were identifying the main factors responsible for health. The rainbow model (Dahlgren & Whitehead, 2021) described a multifactorial approach with layers of both individual and social factors. Layer one includes inherited attributes and genetics, factors associated with age, lifestyle factors like diet and physical activity, and relationships with friends, family and others in the local community. Layer two includes working conditions, housing and access to healthcare. The outermost layer includes socioeconomic conditions, cultural factors and environmental conditions.

There are many other factors, over and above lifestyle factors, involved in health. The Canadian Institute of Advanced Research (2012) (reported in Kuznetsova, 2012) has estimated how much these factors determine health outcomes. They estimate that socioeconomic factors determine 50% of the variation in health, with healthcare determining 25%, the environment determining 15% and genetics determining 10% of health.

These are borne out by the data relating to psoriasis. For example, we know economic hardship plays a role in psoriasis severity (Thomsen et al., 2019), just as it does in health overall. Exposure to environmental pollutants, such as cadmium, also affects psoriasis (Kamiya et al., 2019). In addition, mercury and lead are found in higher levels in the blood of people with psoriasis. It's suggested that these toxins come from food sources and could contribute to inflammation and oxidative stress, an imbalance of free radicals and antioxidants which can cause damage to organs and tissues (Wacewicz-Muczyńska et al., 2021). Certain drugs, like antimalarials, and infections, such as streptococcal throat infections, are well-established factors linked to flare-ups.

Putting diet and lifestyle in perspective

By taking all these factors into account, I can start to adjust my initial belief that diet is the most important determinant. Instead, I can take on board that genetics play a role, as do environmental factors, the efficacy of treatments and waiting lists, etc. Infections probably play a role, as do cuts and scrapes, the weather as well as opportunities to holiday in the sun. When I look at it like this, I can see there is a very small amount that's directly under my control. Appreciating this helps me to feel less blame and self-criticism. Maybe I could allow myself an extra ice-cream on holiday after all.

Summary

- What causes our psoriasis and what makes it flare up is a complex picture without clear answers.
- One thing we do know for sure is that self-blame and self-criticism are unhelpful for emotional well-being.
- Trying to work out what you're doing wrong is a normal reaction to not knowing the underlying causes of psoriasis.
- While improving your lifestyle is a good thing and it will benefit you in numerous ways, regardless of how you eat, what you weigh, how stressed you get, you're not to blame.
- Remember, psoriasis is not your fault.

Top tips

It can help to remind yourself:

- Psoriasis is an immune-mediated inflammatory disease.
- It is not our fault that we developed psoriasis.
- There are multiple factors involved in symptoms and the course of the condition, and most of these are out of an individual's control.
- Having psoriasis does not mean we're not taking care of ourselves.
- Blame and guilt just make us feel badly about ourselves.
- Leading a healthy lifestyle is good for everyone, including those of us with psoriasis.
- Leading a healthy lifestyle may have many benefits regardless of whether it has any impact on our psoriasis.
- We wouldn't blame people with other autoimmune diseases, like coeliac disease, for their conditions, so why blame ourselves?

8   Psoriasis and emotions

> *People often mistake numbness for nothingness, but numbness isn't the absence of feelings;* ***it's a response to being overwhelmed by too many feelings****.*
> — Lori Gottleib (Gottlieb Lori, 2019)

By the time I was 13 years old, psoriasis was raging through my body. I had thick, red flaky patches of skin over my arms, legs and torso. My scalp was crusted with plaques, which flaked into my hair and onto my shoulders. I was prescribed greasy ointments, which stained my clothes and did little apart from softening the plaques. But my life carried on regardless, with school and hobbies, and I joined the supporting cast for our village pantomime, enjoying the fun of rehearsals and learning new songs. It was an annual and much-anticipated event held in the village hall. This year was to be the last time I took part.

It was the night of the opening show, my family had all bought tickets, and I was looking forward to it. The constant itching of my scalp was affecting my sleep and my mood, and I had tried everything from olive oil to coal tar shampoos. Earlier that evening, in desperation for some relief, I took the greasy ointment prescribed for the skin on my body and applied it to my scalp. It felt so soothing, and the thick plaques began to lift and cling to my grease-soaked hair. I got on with my homework, leaving it to work its magic on my scalp and then tried to wash it off. An hour later, it was as greasy as ever. I had tried every shampoo in the house, bars of soap, washing up liquid, and nothing was shifting the grease. All the washing had distributed the flakes of skin from my scalp into my hair, where they held fast, shining white against my dark hair.

I was desperate. I looked terrible and there was no way I wanted to see anyone, let alone stand on a spotlit stage in front of my family, friends and neighbours. Crying, I wanted to stay at home and tell people I was sick. But I felt pressure and didn't want to let anyone down, knowing I would be disappointed in myself after all the hard work and rehearsals. And so I went and performed.

To this day, I feel traumatised by the experience. I don't know if anyone noticed my greasy, psoriasis-flecked hair, but the shame I felt was intense. I couldn't even hide away in the corner of the room. I was exposed on a brightly lit stage for all to scrutinise.

My strategy for coping was to switch off emotionally and numb myself to the terrible feeling of being so out of control. I sang and danced in the background in a robotic fashion and at the end, when everyone crowded around with congratulations, I blocked out all my feelings.

That wasn't the end of the story. An emergency trip to the local hair salon ended in the whole hairdressing team crowding around while the manager gave them a demonstration on how to wash greasy hair. I sat with an audience of stylists all focused on my greasy locks and flaking scalp. Dry-eyed and blank-faced, I stared at the salon ceiling as the manager scrubbed at my scalp and lectured his team. But even his professional shampooing technique didn't work and so as a last resort, they cut my long hair. A few weeks later, the grease had finally come out and by then, the psoriasis on my scalp was as bad as ever but now I also had an unwanted short hairstyle. My coping style, which consisted of closing myself off from pain, shame and despair, had grown in strength. My skin was thickening both literally and metaphorically.

I share this story to help illustrate how the trauma of living with psoriasis, and its uncontrollable nature, teaches you to shut down emotionally. It's as though you switch off from your psoriasis and your shame and stop identifying with it as your own. It feels like a survival strategy.

Alexithymia

Switching off from your internal emotional world is sometimes called alexithymia. In simple terms, alexithymia is a lack of awareness of one's emotional state (or emotional blindness). This might mean someone with alexithymia would struggle to tell whether they were angry, sad or happy. They have difficulty identifying their emotions and describing their emotional state. This extends to finding it hard to differentiate between physical symptoms and emotions; for example, being unable to tell the difference between the sensation of hunger and excitement.

Alexithymia is also linked to a lack of imagination; those with high levels of alexithymia have a limited fantasy world. In particular, they are less likely to spend time imagining positive possibilities or fantasies (Luminet et al., 2000). People with alexithymia tend not to be introspective. They don't spend time wondering how they're feeling and why, and this extends to their interest in other people's emotional worlds; they're unable to identify emotions in others. People who have high levels of alexithymia are often described as lacking in empathy.

When faced with problems, people with alexithymia are more likely to use practical strategies rather than using an emotional approach, like emotional expression or seeking support (Picardi et al., 2005) (Luminet et al., 2000). There's good evidence that telling other people about your emotional state is related to benefits in both mental and physical well-being (Pennebaker et al., 2001). However, people with high levels of alexithymia are less likely to be aware of their emotions, let alone share them with others, leaving them at a disadvantage.

Alexithymia can stop an individual coping appropriately with a stressful life event, since they have limited awareness of their levels of stress and so don't act in other helpful ways to remove or deal with the stressor. Because of this, scientists have suggested that alexithymia may be a trigger for many health conditions, with people not noticing or seeking help for unexplained or worsening symptoms. Indeed, alexithymia is found to be associated with a variety of health conditions including psoriasis, gastrointestinal diseases, pain, cancer and asthma (Figure 8.1).

Research linking alexithymia and psoriasis

Plenty of scientific research has been conducted into the prevalence of alexithymia in people with psoriasis. An early study published in 1998 compared alexithymia in people with psoriasis and three other groups: a control group with no skin condition, people with fungal disease and people with a psychiatric diagnosis of depression or anxiety (Chaudhury

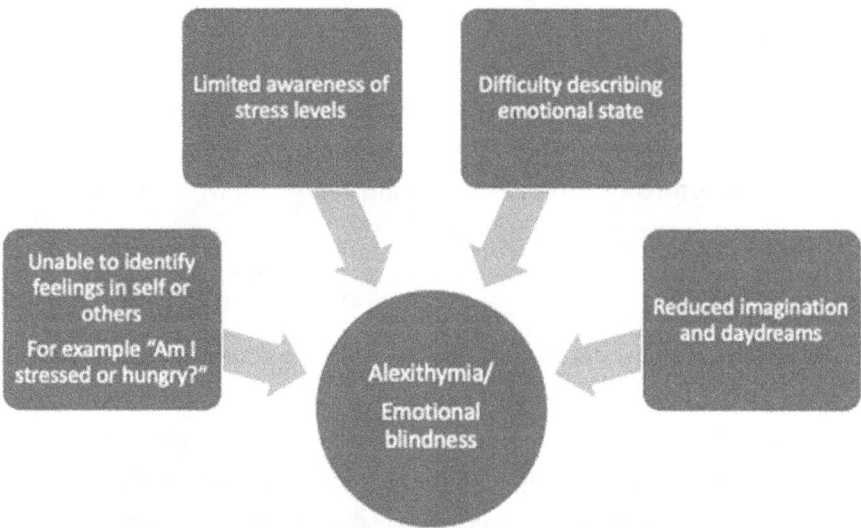

FIGURE 8.1 Traits associated with alexithymia

et al., 1998). They found that levels of alexithymia were higher in people with psoriasis than controls and those hospitalised patients with a fungal infection, but not those with anxiety or depression.

Since that time, there have been numerous studies reporting high rates of alexithymia in psoriasis, generally around a quarter of people with the condition (Tang et al., 2022). The results all suggest the same thing: that people with psoriasis are more prone to emotional blindness. Interestingly, levels of alexithymia don't seem to be linked with gender, age, psoriasis severity or the length of time with the condition (Cherrez-Ojeda et al., 2019). You can find similar rates of alexithymia in other dermatological and health conditions.

There's also evidence to suggest that people with psoriasis have difficulty interpreting facial expressions of disgust (Elise Kleyn et al., 2009). MRI scans were used to look at the insula cortex, the part of the brain that's activated when we see an expression of disgust, in 13 males with psoriasis. They compared the scans with those of males without psoriasis. What they found was that for people with psoriasis, the insula cortex produced much smaller signals in response to facial expressions of disgust. The two groups didn't differ in their brain activity when shown fearful faces or a neutral expression. The difference appeared to be just for expressions of disgust. The scientists argue that by blocking the processing of expressions of disgust, people with psoriasis are protecting themselves against distress. This may relate to previous experiences of being stigmatised.

In a more recent large-scale study spanning 61 centres across 13 countries (Sampogna et al., 2019), people who had been diagnosed with psoriasis in the previous decade completed several questionnaires including the Toronto Alexithymia Scale (TAS-20). They were studied over a year during which time they received phototherapy, systemic or biologic treatment to see whether levels of alexithymia changed in line with other factors. The questionnaires were repeated at six months and one-year points.

The researchers found that, at the start of the study, around a quarter of people scored as having alexithymia, twice as many as were found in the general population. This group was more likely to have a poorer quality of life, to feel depressed and anxious, and to be dependent on alcohol. They were more likely to be out of work, but even when they were in work, they were less productive.

However, people's levels of alexithymia were not fixed. Over time, levels of alexithymia reversed for many, especially if psoriasis severity improved. The biggest changes were seen in people's abilities to identify and describe their feelings. Reversion in alexithymia was associated with big improvements in quality of life, depression and anxiety, and alcohol use. This suggests to me that emotional blindness is a strategy used by many people with psoriasis to cope with the emotional challenges of living with the condition and as the plaques improve, so the defences are lowered.

Coping mechanism vs. personality trait

Alexithymia is often described as a personality trait, meaning it's a built-in part of your character. It's a line of enquiry in psoriasis research that to me has always felt like adding insult to injury. On top of the burden of living with an incurable skin condition, I'm told it's quite likely I also have a defective personality.

I'm not sure how helpful that is to me, other than to add to my already battered self-esteem. As a psychologist, I don't consider this to be a useful personality trait to aid me in my work. But I do recognise times when my psoriasis has been bad, where it has been stressful and I've been feeling low and found it harder to connect with my feelings. For me, this has always been a way of coping with the overwhelming and uncontrollable.

Despite my reticence to embrace this line of scientific research, I can also see how this knowledge could be helpful. Since alexithymia is also observed in people who have experienced adversity in childhood, I prefer to understand some forms of alexithymia as a learnt defence mechanism in response to psoriasis; a condition that is difficult to control and impacts the way the world sees you. The experience I described at the start of this chapter was not the only time I felt traumatised, and I expect the experience of being shamed and exposed is typical for someone with psoriasis. You can't always hide it, especially in childhood when other people are deciding what activities you must participate in and what you should wear, and you can't always shield yourself from other people's expressions of disgust. Over time, you will learn to cope by becoming more alexithymic and distant from painful emotions.

Polyvagal theory

The polyvagal theory is another way to understand how emotional blindness could be a reaction to the trauma of living with psoriasis. According to the theory, the autonomic nervous system, a network of nerves that controls involuntary processes like heart rate, digestion and breathing, constantly monitors the environment, taking account of what's going on in our bodies as well as our surroundings, to check whether things are safe. Much of this happens beneath the level of conscious awareness via neuroception – when faced with danger, the sympathetic branch of the autonomic nervous system is activated, and the fight or flight response is triggered (which we looked at in more detail in Chapter 4).

The parasympathetic nervous system is a branch of the autonomic nervous system that controls involuntary processes designed to relax your body after periods of stress. It triggers two other pathways in response to the environment: the ventral vagal pathway and the dorsal vagal pathway. In the ventral vagal pathway, when the environment is safe, the body does not need to respond to stress or danger, and there is an opportunity for connection with others. In this state, we feel calm and cared for, and we can 'rest and digest'.

When the environment is dangerous and inescapable, the dorsal vagal pathway activates instead. This pathway gets us to respond by immobilisation, not only emotionally but also physically, shutting down bodily systems to preserve energy. It's the 'playing dead' response we might observe in some animals, like the possum, when under threat. In a dorsal vagal state, we freeze and feel numb and we pull away from connection with others. Due to less oxygen flow to the brain, it can result in a feeling of absence or dissociation. There's evidence that many people faced with inescapable trauma dissociate from the experience.

Stephen Porges (Porges, 2009), who proposed the polyvagal theory, describes how the autonomic nervous system reacts to stress by moving a person between states. Dana (2018) describes it as being like a ladder with ventral vagal at the top and a person moving down to the next rung: sympathetic/flight or fight, and if that doesn't resolve the threat then as a last resort moving to dorsal vagal where the person shuts down. A person goes through the stages as if they were climbing down a ladder, and when in dorsal vagal, a person needs to go through sympathetic before climbing back to ventral vagal (Figure 8.2).

Proponents of the polyvagal theory suggest that people who have experienced trauma may have a misaligned neuroceptive system, leading the nervous system to perceive danger where there is none, for example being triggered by the sound of a siren or the sight of a symbol relating to the trauma, like a red coat or a particular scent. This leads the nervous system to move rapidly through sympathetic to dorsal vagal and people can switch off and dissociate at a trigger. It's certainly

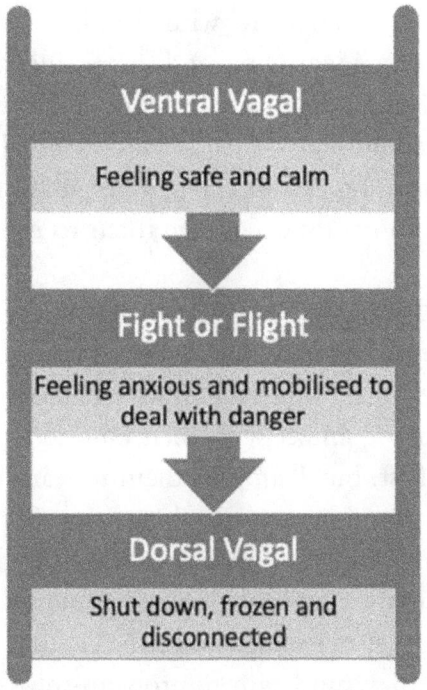

FIGURE 8.2 Polyvagal theory. Source: Adapted from Dana, 2018

possible that people with psoriasis rapidly move to the dorsal vagal in situations that have been previously traumatising or stigmatising, resulting in emotional numbness.

Alexithymia and depression

People who are depressed also show high rates of alexithymia, leading some people to question whether alexithymia is in fact a symptom of depression rather than a separate construct. In her memoir, psychotherapist Lori Gottlieb (Gottlieb, 2019) describes how easy it is to mistake 'numbness' for an absence of emotions when instead it's due to overwhelming feelings. She argues that shutting down and pulling away from emotional pain can be a coping response to trauma that can mask the expression of low mood and depression.

In my job as a psychologist, I often work with people who are depressed and who have difficulty identifying and expressing their emotions. A large part of the therapy I do is to help people have better insight and awareness of their emotional world. It's not unusual for someone to tell me about a distressing experience in a very flat, non-emotional way, and it's my job to gently encourage them to explore their related feelings.

At first, when people are struggling to recognise their emotions, I start by suggesting how I imagine I would feel if I'd been through the same experience as them. Some of the most important therapy I do with people is to help them really connect with their emotions. For most people, this feels scary at first, but I support them to learn that though they may be powerful, emotions are not dangerous. Slowly, people start to notice and listen to the emotional signals their body is sending them, which is an important step in their healing journey. As people begin to understand how they're feeling and learn that they can cope with their emotions, then they can begin to problem-solve and work towards ways of resolving their difficulties.

There's good evidence that alexithymia can change with psychotherapy, which would suggest that it's not a fixed personality trait. In a review of 23 studies looking at psychotherapy in various populations of people with high levels of alexithymia (Cameron et al., 2014), the authors conclude that alexithymia can be changed, with many studies reporting significant reductions. In several studies, the changes in levels of alexithymia paralleled improvements in depression. Such psychotherapy typically includes exercises like practising communication skills and non-verbal body language, recording dreams and focusing attention on internal experiences.

Strategies to deal with emotional blindness

Although I know there are times when I shut down emotionally, I don't identify with the signs of high alexithymia. However, given that countless research studies have identified higher rates of alexithymia in people with psoriasis, you might be interested to know whether you are one of those people with high levels. There are questionnaires you can use like the Toronto Alexithymia Scale (TAS-20) (Bagby et al., 1994). This asks about three possible dimensions of alexithymia and produces a score which will tell you how you are in comparison to others.

Dimensions of the Toronto Alexithymia Scale

Difficulty identifying feelings

Being confused about what emotion you're feeling.
   Feeling puzzled by sensations in your body.
   Not knowing why you're feeling angry.

Difficulty describing feelings

Not being able to find the right words to describe the way you're feeling.
   Finding it hard to describe how you feel about people.
   Finding it difficult to talk about your innermost feelings, even with your friends and family.

Externally orientated thinking

Preferring to talk to people about what they've been doing rather than what they've been feeling.
   Not to find it particularly helpful to examine your feelings when solving a problem.
   Not needing to analyse why things turned out the way they did.

If you think you have higher levels of alexithymia or emotional blindness, then there are things you can do to increase your ability to identify your own and other people's feelings.

Keeping a diary can be a good starting point. As you write about things that happened during your day, try to remember how it felt at the time. Was it a nice feeling? Did you laugh? Were you happy?

This might be tricky at first, but it will get easier with practise. If you are writing an entry about other people, try to identify how they were feeling too. Note down how their body and facial expression looked (e.g. was it tense, were they smiling?). If you struggle with this, perhaps you could ask them. You might remember to ask them at the time knowing that you'll want to write about it later, or if it's someone who knows you're keeping the diary, you could always ask them later. You could create a list of the most common emotions and their descriptions to keep alongside your diary. You can start with the five core emotions: happiness, fear, sadness, disgust and anger. Build your list as you start to explore emotions. Humans can experience many different emotions. Some scientists have even suggested it's as many as 34,000 (Plutchik, 1980), so that's a lot to choose from. If you're struggling to think of many different emotions, you could try searching for lists of emotions online.

Reading fictional novels can also help. As you're reading, try to focus on the emotions of the characters. Authors don't always tell us directly how someone is feeling, but you can pick up clues from the text. Is the character's heart beating fast? Are they gripping their pen tight, and so on? Consider joining a book club where you can discuss the characters, their motives and emotions with others. It will be good to get other people's viewpoints too.

You can also try a minute of mindfulness at the start, middle and end of your day. Take a moment to focus your attention on your breathing and then notice how you're feeling. Are your shoulders tense, is your forehead creased up, do you have butterflies in your tummy? It will help to have regular check-ins like this and ask yourself, how am I feeling right now?

Why not try a hobby that involves emotional expression such as dancing or acting? Acting can be especially useful by getting yourself into character and imagining how you should behave to show an audience how you are feeling. When you're watching a movie or the television, notice what emotions the actors are portraying and how they're doing that. If you're watching with someone who doesn't mind talking over a film, ask them what they think the actors are feeling too.

Therapy, in particular Interpersonal Psychotherapy (IPT), can be helpful in learning to become more aware of your emotions. IPT can also help you mentalise or put yourself in other people's shoes and understand their emotions too. Typically, IPT therapists will use a range of strategies like role play to help someone learn to mentalise.

Summary

- Scientists have found that people with psoriasis tend to have high levels of alexithymia.
- Alexithymia is an inability to identify emotions in yourself and others.
- People who have experienced trauma or who are depressed also have high levels of alexithymia.
- Being able to identify emotions is important for physical and mental health.
- In psoriasis, alexithymia reduces when the skin is treated effectively.
- Alexithymia can also change with psychological therapy.

Top tips

- Start to take an interest in your emotional world.
- Even when it feels powerful, remind yourself that your emotions are not dangerous.
- Knowing how you're feeling emotionally can help you get the right support at the right time.

9 Relationships and intimacy

> *If he could learn to love another, and earn her love in return by the time the last petal fell, then the spell would be broken. If not, he would be doomed to remain a beast for all time. As the years passed, he fell into despair and lost all hope. For who could ever learn to love a beast?*
>
> — *Beauty and the Beast*, © Disney

Having psoriasis affects your relationships and the way you interact with people, which can have consequences for your physical and mental health, and make you more vulnerable in times of crisis. Just like the Beast who hides in his castle afraid of the way people might react to his appearance, there have been times when I've isolated myself from others and my instinct has always been to hide my skin. I've had to work really hard to be able to look at my reflection in a compassionate manner. It comes much easier to me to gaze upon my reflection with disgust. I hate the way the inflamed and flaky patches are scattered across my body. At times, I felt like a monster and wondered who could ever find me attractive.

Social distancing

Psoriasis can make us less willing to socialise, date and make friends, leading to withdrawal and isolation.

I have always been fearful of what people would think of me if they saw my skin at its worst. My fear has led me to hide away, and I have turned down many invitations. I've never been tempted to join friends for a spa day, and I've avoided going away to conferences if it meant I would have to share a hotel room with a colleague.

Having psoriasis has meant that I have kept people at a distance at times, fearful of revealing my skin and flakes. For those with psoriatic arthritis (PsA), there are additional difficulties associated with accessing many activities. Many people with the condition have trouble doing activities that involve lots of walking, climbing stairs or standing, and this can put further limits on opportunities to interact with others and form bonds.

Relationships

Dating with psoriasis is particularly difficult. Luckily, I met my husband soon after a course of phototherapy and I was tanned and clear. By the time the plaques had returned, I trusted in his devotion to me, but even so I've always struggled to believe that I look attractive to him.

The American writer John Updike felt the same way about his closest relationships. At the time he was writing *From the Journal of a Leper* (Updike, John, 1985) his psoriasis was severe, and he was due to start phototherapy with assurances of clearance from his doctor. He shared this news with his girlfriend:

> *I told Carlotta tonight of his casual promise to make me 'clear'. She says she loves me the way I am. 'How can you!' I blurt. She shrugs.*

As the treatment began to work, he became offended by Carlotta's celebration of his clearing skin. Emboldened by his recovery, she told him she had previously worried about hurting him when she touched his skin and was also startled to wake in the morning covered in his flakes of skin. Her confession distressed Updike:

> *I had dared dream I was beautiful, if not in her eyes and to her touch, then in her heart, in the glowing heart of her love. But even there, I see now, I was a leper.*

Navigating intimacy

Like Updike, many people with psoriasis are cautious about engaging in intimate relationships. A poor body image, feelings of shame, discomfort, pain, stress and anxiety can all affect libido and the desire to be intimate.

With up to 63% of people with psoriasis having plaques and lesions on their genital areas at some point during the course of their condition (Yang et al., 2018), and skin and joint pain which can lead to discomfort during sexual activity (Snyder et al., 2022), it's not surprising that the majority of us feel reluctant to date at all (Anstey et al., 2012).

You may feel so embarrassed about having psoriasis in intimate areas that you're reluctant to mention it to your doctor and leave it untreated. If this is the case, remind yourself that so many of us experience psoriasis in the genital area and your doctor won't be shocked or even surprised. Treatments for those parts of your body can be different from other areas, so it's important to address it and get the right help.

Being touched

Psoriasis can lead to the avoidance of touch in both platonic and intimate relationships with the fear that someone's fingers will brush against a plaque and they'll recoil. I've always hated anyone placing their hand on the back of my neck, a part of my body often encrusted with psoriasis and usually hidden by my hair. Avoiding touch can have negative consequences. Touch is not only an important way of communicating in a close or intimate relationship, but it's also linked with the release of the hormone oxytocin, known as the love hormone, which gives you a warm, fuzzy feeling and helps strengthen bonds with others. Touch has positive physical effects too; it can calm us, slow our heart rate and reduce blood pressure.

Sadly, touch has different connotations for people with psoriasis who not only feel negative about touching their own skin but also report less pleasure from being touched by anyone; even cuddles from parents are evaluated as negative (Lahousen et al., 2014).

Contrary to what you might expect, in intimate relationships, people with psoriasis tend to appraise the experience of being touched by a partner as more pleasurable. The researchers suggest that 'psoriasis patients, who are in a relationship, tend to idealise their relationship, because they are thankful for having found a partner who accepts him/her despite the affected skin' (Lahousen et al., 2014). I'm not sure whether this is true for me, but when someone touches me, my attention is usually drawn to my psoriasis rather than the experience of being touched.

Interpersonal skills

Having psoriasis can impact interpersonal skills, which might make building relationships more difficult. Alexithymia or emotional blindness (discussed in the previous chapter) triggered by stress and trauma can mean an individual doesn't know how they're feeling and so can't express that. As a result, they are less likely to engage with others.

In addition, growing up with feelings of shame in childhood and adolescence can lead to aggression in the face of criticism. Evidence suggests that children who feel higher levels of shame are viewed as less empathic and less popular than their peers, and the way they manage their anger is seen as less constructive (Tangney et al., 1996). Someone who is prone to shame as an adult may respond to criticism with defensiveness and denial, even when the criticism is constructive. This, in turn has implications for how people respond back to them, leading to problems in developing and maintaining relationships. Evidence suggests that people with psoriasis tend to have an avoidant attachment style, where they resist closeness and intimacy, leading to reduced emotional closeness and intimacy in relationships (Picardi et al., 2005).

Loneliness

We strive to hide our skin and avoid being seen. This leads us to withdraw from situations and other people, but it's not a helpful long-term coping strategy. Not feeling seen is a lonely state to be in.

According to the World Psoriasis Happiness Report (2018), around a quarter of women and a fifth of men with psoriasis experience loneliness (Leo Innovation Lab and Happiness Research Institute, 2018).

Loneliness can raise levels of stress hormones and inflammation, which in turn can increase the risk of chronic illness such as heart disease and type 2 diabetes. There's good evidence of increased rates of sleep disruption, abnormal immune responses and accelerated cognitive decline among socially isolated people (Khullar, 2016).

The people we have in our lives, the ways in which we are connected to others and the quality of our relationships are important determinants of someone's physical and mental health. The Harvard study of Adult Development tracked the lives of over 700 men from the general population over their teenage years into old age. They gathered a lot of information about these men's lives: their health, their work, their income and their relationships. Happiness for these men was not linked to wealth, fame or success at work. The overwhelming finding was that good connections with family, friends and community kept men happier and healthier. In contrast, those men who were more isolated than they wanted to be were less healthy, less happy and more likely to die younger. The quality of connections was also shown to be important with warm relationships having a protective impact on health and longevity.

The importance of social relationships

People who lack close and supportive relationships are more vulnerable in times of crisis or stress. Not only that, but social relationships are literally lifesaving. There are numerous studies confirming that relationships predict mortality. A range of studies following more than 300,000 people over several years found that those with fewer social relationships were more likely to die regardless of their age, gender and health at the start of the study (Holt-Lunstad et al., 2010). The lack of relationships is a risk of similar magnitude to smoking, and bigger than other risk factors associated with mortality such as obesity and physical inactivity.

In my clinical practice, regardless of the nature of the difficulties someone presents with, I find it helpful to understand an individual's social network. I ask about the different people in someone's life and consider the strength and quality of the relationships. I'm also interested in how my client relates to others. Do they find it difficult to accept help? Are they trusting? Do they try hard to please others? Are they able to put themselves in someone else's shoes? All these things are important in developing relationships and accessing support from friends and family.

Different types of social support

For your emotional well-being, it's helpful to have relationships that provide different types of support in your life:

- Emotional support: these are the people we can rely on in a crisis, who can give us a shoulder to cry on. This kind of support is particularly important if you're feeling low in mood or anxious.
- Practical support: we also need people who can offer practical help like collecting children from school if you get stuck at work or helping with laundry if your washing machine breaks.
- Enjoyable support: it's important to have people you can have fun with, who lift your spirits and whom you enjoy being around.
- Cheerleader support: this is provided by people who can encourage you or help you achieve things of importance to you (Figure 9.1).

You may be lucky enough to have people in your life who fulfil all of these functions, but it's more common to have a network of relationships with a range of different people who fulfil various needs. Having psoriasis might mean that you have fewer relationships and so there's a chance that you don't have all of these types of support, which can make life more difficult.

If you're anything like me, spending most of your life hiding psoriasis and ignoring it, then that results in avoiding telling people when it's a struggle. I keep my tears and my worries to myself, which is

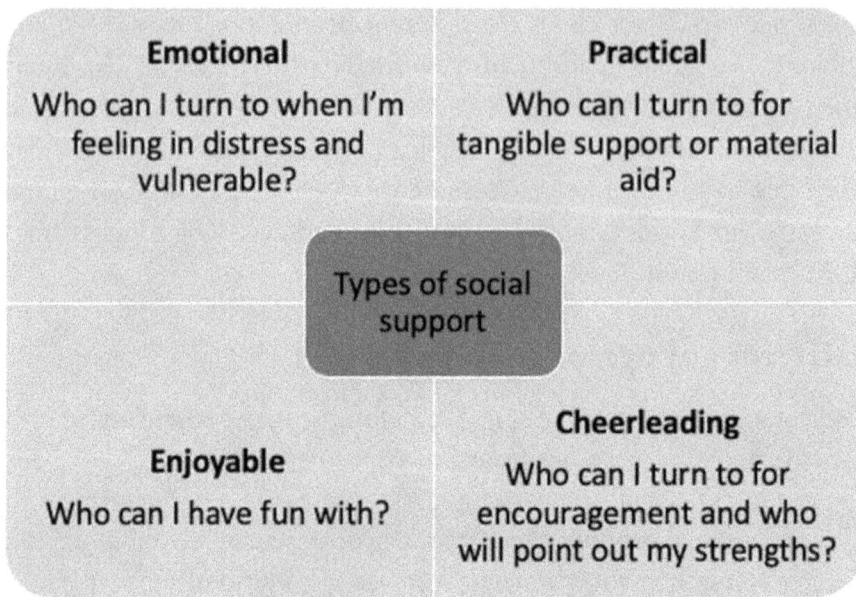

FIGURE 9.1 Different types of social support

not especially helpful. While I tell myself that there's no point sharing my struggles with others as it won't make any difference to the psoriasis, I am missing the point of sharing my emotional world with others. The research evidence tells me I'm not alone in this: people with more severe psoriasis are also less likely to seek social support (Scharloo et al., 2000).

Sharing your emotions

Although sharing emotions won't have any impact on the severity of my skin or cure me, it is helpful to talk to someone who is empathetic and supportive because it will make me feel better. I will feel understood by my friends and family and I won't feel so alone. I will feel validated about my feelings and experiences.

By acknowledging and talking through my emotions, I can begin to understand the difficulties and I can start to problem-solve and think about the little things that might make a difference. 'A problem shared is a problem halved' is an age-old saying, but talking about your feelings can really help you to feel and cope better.

Not only that, but relationships are deepened when you reach out to someone and ask for help. There's good evidence that we feel more connected to people, and we value the relationship more, if someone has asked us to do something for them. I know I like to be able to do things for my friends. It makes me feel good about myself and it reminds me how much I care for them. Reciprocity, being able to give support and receive support, is a crucial part of relationship building and you're denying your friends the chance to reciprocate if you never open up and ask for help.

> ### Try this
>
> If you're not used to talking about your difficulties, it can be difficult to know how to start a conversation, let alone ask for help. Having some conversation openers prepared can be useful. For example:
>
> *I had my clinic appointment today, have you got five minutes to talk about it?*
>
> *I'm trying to find an outfit to wear to my sister's wedding and it's been really hard because I want to hide my psoriasis. Do you have time for a coffee and talk it through?*

If you've started to wonder whether having psoriasis has affected your relationships, then it might be worth considering the following questions:

Who do I have in my life right now?
Am I satisfied with the number of people I'm connected to and the quality of those relationships?
Do I get different types of support from my relationships? Is something missing?

Is there give-and-take in my relationships?
Do I share how I'm feeling emotionally?
Who can I talk to about my struggles with psoriasis?

Strengthening relationships

If you recognise that you could have better support around you, or you lack close and fulfilling relationships, there are things you can do to strengthen relationships. Reach out to people by sending a text or an email and suggest meeting up or spending time doing something you both enjoy. Arrange to spend quality time with them away from the pressures of everyday family or work life.

Sometimes we let friendships drift as life gets busy, and we fail to stay in touch. If this has happened to you, then you may be able to rekindle the relationship by getting in touch online, by phone or even an old-fashioned letter. You could arrange to catch up in person.

If you think you'd like to make new friends, then research what local activities or groups are available where you might meet like-minded people. For example, if you love reading, perhaps your local library has a book group or if film is a passion, maybe there's a nearby community cinema where you could volunteer.

There may be other opportunities in your life right now to connect with people. Perhaps you could start eating your lunch in the work staff room rather than sitting at your desk, or join in with the next work social rather than automatically giving your apologies.

It might feel awkward at first, and it certainly takes courage to do something different, but I believe that developing and strengthening your relationships will help you to cope with your psoriasis.

The dating game

Dating with psoriasis takes a great deal of courage. Even actress and model Cara Delevingne has reported problems dating due to her psoriasis. Knowing when or how to talk about your psoriasis can be tricky. If you can hide your psoriasis with clothes or make-up, then you might not want to talk about it on a first or second date. That's perfectly fine, but at some point, if the relationship becomes more serious, you'll need to open up and explain about your skin. This will seem scary, so have what you're going to say prepared and practise with a friend. Don't be afraid to change the subject if you've had enough of talking about it. But if the person you're dating wants to know more, you could point them in the direction of some good reputable websites (see recommended sites in the Appendix at the end of the book).

Remind yourself about all the qualities that someone might find attractive in you. If you find that difficult, make a list of the things you are attracted to in a person and order them in terms of importance. For me, the top attributes in a partner would be kindness, sense of humour, intelligence, whether we share the same interests. What their skin looks like would not feature on my list. When you have your list, ask yourself, why it is you think on everyone else's list skin would be one of the most important attributes? Personally, I wouldn't want to date someone who lists perfect skin as one of the most important characteristics they're looking for in a partner. If someone doesn't want to date you because you don't have perfect skin, you've probably dodged a bullet.

Accepting praise about your appearance

If, like me, you struggle to believe someone when they tell you they find you attractive, then there are things you can do to help with this. Most of the time we're trying to be psoriasis mind readers, assuming what people are thinking about us and believing what they're saying isn't true. We easily discount any evidence that contradicts our deep-seated beliefs of being unattractive, but we're on the lookout for any slithers of evidence that confirms our negative view of how we look. You can read more about how our thinking impacts the way we feel about ourselves in Chapter 12.

Reclaiming touch

Just because you have psoriasis, you needn't miss out on the basic pleasure of being touched. If you've avoided touch for a long time, now is the time to do something different and feel better about it. It could even start with moisturising. Applying moisturiser for me is just another treatment. I don't miss a day of applying my thick prescribed non-perfumed cream everywhere. As an aside, my children all love the smell of one particular prescription moisturiser. It's non-perfumed and doesn't smell all that great to me, but when they smell it, it reminds them of me and brings them comfort.

There's nothing luxurious or pampering about my prescription moisturiser, so from time to time I use an expensive body cream and I apply it in a mindful way, enjoying the scent and the relaxing sensation of massaging it into my skin. I slow my breathing; I feel the ointment on my fingers and the palms of my hands, I pay attention to the temperature of my skin, and how it feels as I massage the cream in.

When my attention is drawn to psoriasis as it inevitably is, I try to notice it's there without judgement rather than get into a stream of inner conversation about how bad it is, how awful it looks and so on. This is not an easy task, but every time my mind gets pulled away from the scent and the feel of the cream, I notice I've become distracted and turn my attention back to the cream. This might happen a couple of times or fifty times. I don't get frustrated with myself. Instead, I refocus on the smell and texture of the cream as I rub it into my skin. In this small way, I am retraining myself to enjoy the sensation of touch despite psoriasis.

A mindful massage could be an activity you do with a partner. Ask them to read this chapter so they understand how difficult it can be to enjoy touch when you have psoriasis. Then suggest they give you a massage. You could start somewhere where you know the psoriasis isn't so bad, like your back or shoulders, and at first just try a massage for a short amount of time. Try to practise the same mindful attention to the feeling of being touched and just as I described above, when you focus on your psoriasis, try not to get into an internal debate with yourself about whether your partner has felt it. Instead, notice that your attention has wandered and then bring it back to the massage.

An alternative would be to book a professional massage. Before your appointment, call up and explain that you have psoriasis and discuss your options. As a professional, they will be used to seeing all kinds of skin types and should have a good understanding about psoriasis. Word of mouth can be a great way to find a masseur who is used to working with people with psoriasis.

Connecting with other people with psoriasis

Finally, it's important to build relationships with other people who have psoriasis, and in the days of social media, this couldn't be easier. When I was growing up, one of my best friends also had psoriasis, and even now, we regularly talk about it and swap tips. It's always so comforting because I know she just gets it, and I don't feel so alone. Knowing how stylish and attractive she is, in spite of her psoriasis, helps me challenge my beliefs about how my own psoriasis impacts my appearance. You may also have friends or family with psoriasis, but if you don't know anyone currently, you can meet people by joining online support forums (details listed in the Appendix), and there may be in-person support groups locally to you.

We know it's important to spend time with other people who also have psoriasis because the benefits are numerous: feeling understood, sharing tips and ideas, and meeting other people who are leading happy and fulfilling lives despite their psoriasis. It's a powerful reminder that we're all much more than skin.

When you live with a chronic illness, your relationships are so important, but the very nature of the illness often means it's more difficult to make and sustain them. Putting effort into strengthening and building bonds will make a difference. Those of us lucky enough to have warm relationships live longer, stay healthier and are happier. If all this hasn't convinced you of the importance of relationships, then watch the powerful TED talk by Robert Waldinger, the fourth director of the Harvard Study of Adult Development. He talks about the longest study on happiness and the importance of social connections, and concludes, 'It turns out that people who are more socially connected to family, to friends, to community, are happier, they're physically healthier, and they live longer than people who are less well connected'.

Summary

- People with psoriasis often avoid people and situations due to fear of exposure.
- This avoidance can lead to loneliness and isolation.
- Strong, positive relationships are important for physical and mental well-being.
- Your support network can help you cope with psoriasis.
- There are lots of things you can do to help build relationships.

Top tips

- Think about who you have in your life and how they support you.
- Strengthen existing relationships or look for opportunities to make new ones.
- Share how you feel with those you trust.
- Reach out to other people with psoriasis.
- Take small steps to enjoy touch again.

10 Models of illness beliefs

Bring together a group of people with psoriasis, and while we'll have an awful lot in common, the way we cope with our condition will vary from person to person.

Regardless of how bad their skin is, some people will have great self-esteem, others will feel bad about themselves; some will be very low in mood and others extremely happy. It's part of the reason that support groups and online forums are so helpful. People give advice from their own experiences, and you get to hear a wide range of opinions and beliefs.

In studies looking at quality of life in people with psoriasis, there's always a wide range of responses which can't be completely explained by disease severity. Some people will have a few plaques and report having a poor quality of life, while other people with extensive plaques and joint pain report a good quality of life.

Differing reactions

As a psychologist, it always interests me why people react so differently to illness and threats to health. I'm interested to know why some people seem to be more resilient, some are better at completing their treatments, and some seem not to be distressed by their condition, even at its worst.

I'm also interested to know what makes some people vulnerable to mental health difficulties like depression and anxiety. As someone who works with people with health conditions, it's important to understand the psychological factors that help someone cope so that I can help others.

The study of health behaviour

There's not a straightforward answer to why people respond and cope in such varying ways. We've understood for a long time that the way someone responds to illness is due to a complex mix of biological, social and psychological influences, from the genes you were born with to the community in which you grew up and the decisions you make. The study of health behaviour is fascinating, and research since the 1960s has helped us to understand how people respond to information about their health.

Back in the 1970s, a group of psychologists from Yale University led by Dr Howard Leventhal was studying how individuals respond to, and cope with, health threats. They interviewed people with chronic illnesses, those with a new diagnosis of cancer as well as healthy adults. They discovered a three-step problem-solving model that is largely based on the beliefs an individual holds about that illness: what they believe caused it, what consequences they think it will have and how long they think it will last (Leventhal et al., 1980) (Figure 10.1).

The first step in this problem-solving model is noticing that something is different from the norm and how things usually are. As a child, my first few patches of psoriasis were either mislabelled or brushed off as insignificant; something that I thought would clear up on its own just as other cuts and scrapes had. But as the plaques increased in number and size, I knew something wasn't right. My understanding of skin was that it should be smooth and unbroken and a graze or a scab should heal within a matter of days. But these plaques were very different. I'd never seen psoriasis before, so I didn't understand what it was or how to label it.

In order to know what to do next, I needed to generate a set of beliefs about psoriasis, to guide me in how to respond and react. Within this step in the model, people who've noticed something isn't quite right start to develop an understanding of what's going on. These fall into five categories of beliefs about the illness:

Models of illness beliefs

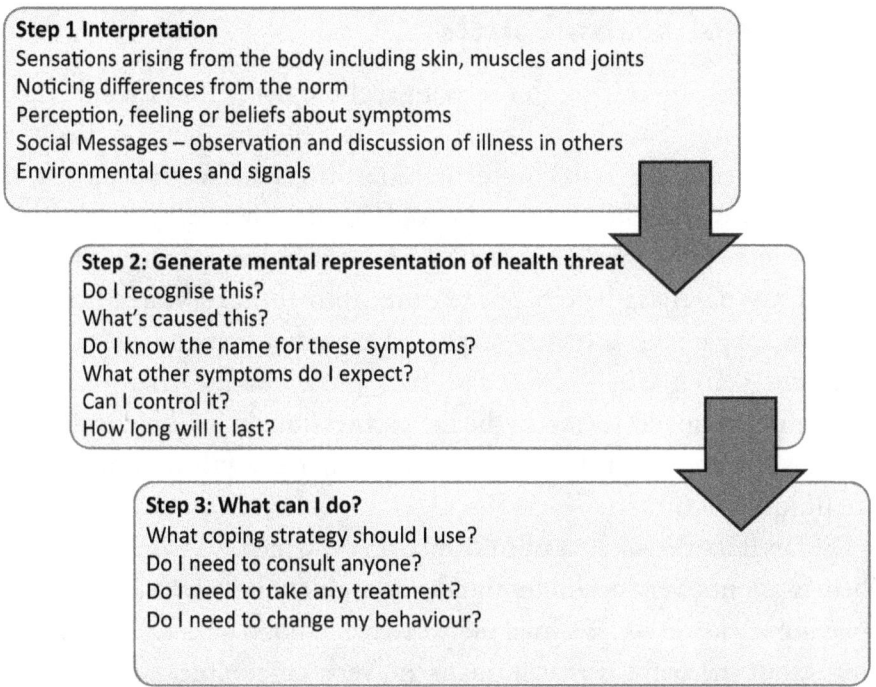

FIGURE 10.1 Three-step problem-solving model. Source: Adapted from Leventhal et al., 1980.

1. Identity – this is the label I give my condition and the symptoms I think go along with it.
2. Cause – these are my beliefs about what caused my condition. They could include my beliefs that it was caused by stress, or by my genetics or by the environment.
3. Timeline – these are my beliefs about how long I think it will last.
4. Consequences – my beliefs about the impact of the condition on my life and well-being.
5. Cure/controllability – my beliefs about whether there is anything I can do to control or cure it.

Sources of health beliefs

What's most interesting to me as a psychologist is that these beliefs are often not based on objective evidence but develop from a variety of sources. This might include things we've read on social media, information we've been told by health professionals and our friends and family, as well as our own lived experiences. A lot of my psoriasis beliefs have come from things I've read online and in magazines and newspapers. I expect for many people, an internet search will provide the first pieces of information. The information given to me by health professionals is likely to be far more accurate, but I don't always remember everything I'm told in a clinic appointment.

Sometimes the sources of information on which we base our illness beliefs are not very accurate. In addition, our minds are very good at playing tricks on us. We imagine we're really good at detecting symptoms, but the truth is that humans are very suggestible, and our perception of symptoms is based on many factors. I've always believed I'm very sensitive to cleaning products, hairspray and perfumes. If, for example, someone were to spray a bathroom cleaner near me, I would itch all over. However, one time when I was watching television, an advert came on for a cleaning product. It was sprayed liberally over the on-screen bathroom, and I reacted instantly by itching. Even though it was obvious to me that the product was having no direct contact with my skin, I still had a physical reaction to it.

Another study in the 1970s (Ruble, 1977) took blood samples from a group of women and from that told them when they were likely to get their period. Then the researchers asked the women to rate their levels of premenstrual symptoms (PMS) like water retention. Women who thought their period was due imminently reported higher levels of PMS. What the researchers didn't tell them was that the estimation of their cycle was completely random. This doesn't mean the symptoms were simply in their head. Instead, it's a complex mix of expectation and attention.

This phenomenon can also be seen in a surprisingly large number of medical students who develop symptoms of the condition they're studying at that time. Known as medical students' disease, this arises due to an increase in knowledge and understanding which leads a student to notice a 'symptom' they would have previously ignored and misattribute it to the illness. It's also likely that medical students develop a level of heightened awareness of the part of the body they are studying as well as a heightened level of anxiety about developing the condition, all of which contribute to the perception of symptoms.

Cultural influences

Our beliefs are also likely to be heavily influenced by the culture in which we live. In the Western world, we tend to follow a medical model where we talk about specialists and experts fighting against illness and infection. Our understanding of ill health is phrased in terms like battles and defences. Many of us are still influenced by earlier beliefs of our ancestors about health requiring balance, for example keeping warm to protect against a cold. There are a range of different cultural beliefs, including spiritual and supernatural forces, from across the world that determine how people understand their illness.

Some of our beliefs about psoriasis will be accurate and lead us to make good decisions, but there's a good chance many will be inaccurate, even our perception of the symptoms we have. Because we hold them implicitly, we don't ever stop to really think about them in detail or to question them. We act on our beliefs, nonetheless. In some situations, our beliefs mislead us, and then we can behave in ways that are not so helpful to our health outcomes.

Acting on our beliefs

Once we have a set of beliefs and an understanding that make sense to us, the next step is how we deal with psoriasis. The different ways of coping we might adopt are directly linked to our beliefs. If I believe that I will never have clear skin no matter what I do, that having psoriasis isn't going to make any difference to my life, and that all treatments are more hassle than they're worth, then I'm unlikely to follow my dermatologist's instructions and use my creams twice a day.

On the other hand, if I believe that psoriasis will ruin my life and if I also believe that I can achieve clear skin if I try hard enough, I will keep pursuing new treatments until I reach that goal.

Evaluating what works

The final step in the problem-solving model is evaluating whether what I've done has worked. If I believe gluten is responsible for my psoriasis, after a while I might start to question why my skin is getting worse even though I've given up gluten. Following this, I will change my beliefs based on my experience and try a different approach.

In this model, a person continually evaluates whether their coping strategies have been effective, adjusting how they cope as they acquire new beliefs through experience and other sources in an attempt to reach a place where their beliefs fit with their experiences.

As before, this isn't an explicit process and not something a person will stop to question. For example, if I'm not expecting my psoriasis to be sore or have a big impact on my life then I need to either adjust my beliefs or what I'm doing if my expectations are wrong. It might be that I'm not using any creams and I've stopped exercising because of the pain, which is making me miserable. Then I might adjust my beliefs slightly, recognising that psoriasis does have an impact on my life after all, and I might try something different like making a doctor's appointment, getting advice online or changing my diet. An alternative belief, that having psoriasis means I can't exercise, might make me feel hopeless and low in mood.

Leventhal and his team of researchers suggested that a person would keep going through the three stages in a process of learning new information, discarding old information, changing beliefs and trying new coping strategies until a status quo is reached, where the individual judges that their coping strategies are effective and the experience of living with the illness fits with their perceptions of that condition (Figure 10.2).

The impact of health beliefs on coping and quality of life

The beliefs you have about illness, regardless of how accurate they are, determine what you do and how you cope, and many researchers have explored this further in psoriasis. A research study (Scharloo et al., 2000) looked at 69 people's beliefs about their psoriasis and whether they predicted how someone would be coping a year later. They found that when people believed they could cure or control their psoriasis, they were more likely to attend clinic appointments. Severity of skin, on the other hand, didn't determine the number of times someone attended a clinic. Interestingly, whether a person believed they were healthy wasn't related to the severity of their psoriasis.

The belief that psoriasis has many negative consequences was related to perceived health. So, if you felt there would be lots of negative consequences caused by psoriasis, then you would be more likely to rate yourself as having poor health regardless of how much of your skin was covered in psoriasis.

A larger study carried out in Turkey with over 300 people with psoriasis found that when people believed they could keep their psoriasis under control and felt they understood it, they had a better quality of life. In this study, people who believed psoriasis was caused by something they did were more likely to have a poor quality of life (Solmaz et al., 2021).

When I was training, I elected to study illness beliefs in psoriasis. I was studying at the University of London and my research supervisor was Professor John Weinman, a leading expert in the field of illness beliefs. My research found that when people believed their psoriasis was caused by stress, they were much more likely to be anxious or depressed than if they thought psoriasis was caused by factors out of

COPING WITH PSORIASIS

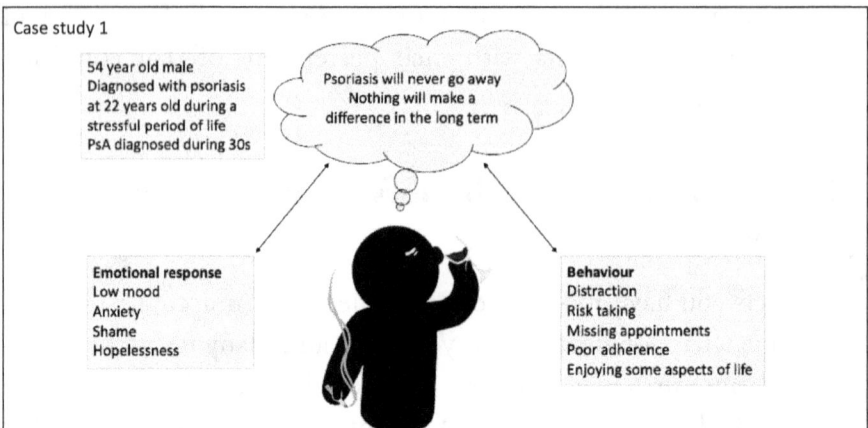

Case study 1

54 year old male
Diagnosed with psoriasis at 22 years old during a stressful period of life
PsA diagnosed during 30s

Thought: Psoriasis will never go away Nothing will make a difference in the long term

Emotional response
Low mood
Anxiety
Shame
Hopelessness

Behaviour
Distraction
Risk taking
Missing appointments
Poor adherence
Enjoying some aspects of life

In the first example, a 54-year-old man has been living with psoriasis and psoriatic arthritis (PsA) since his early twenties. During this time developed lots of beliefs about psoriasis. These include the belief that it will never go away and will always have a big impact on his life. He believes no treatment will make any difference in the long term. Instead of attending appointments or using his treatments, which he believes is ultimately futile, he tries to take his mind off having psoriasis by drinking and through lots of risky behaviour like substance use. He certainly enjoys some aspects of his life, but his health is poor and he feels hopeless about things changing. This leads to feelings of depression and anxiety. He feels ashamed that he's missed so many appointments and his bathroom cabinets are full of unopened prescriptions, so he avoids contact with health professionals.

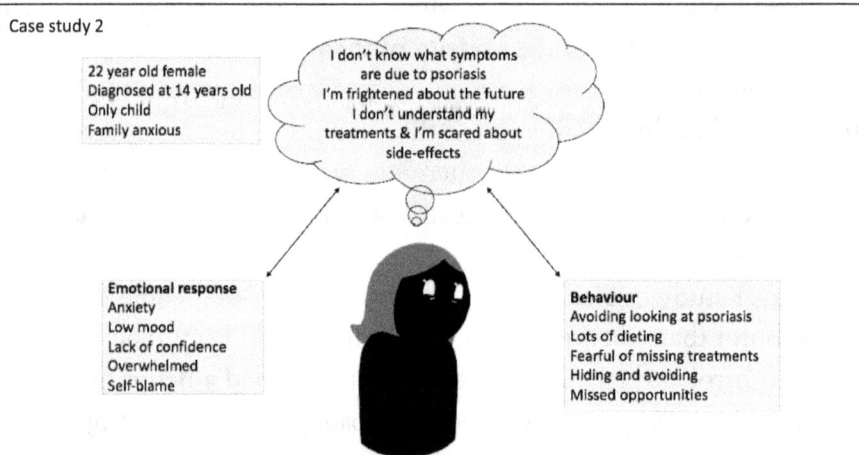

Case study 2

22 year old female
Diagnosed at 14 years old
Only child
Family anxious

Thought: I don't know what symptoms are due to psoriasis
I'm frightened about the future
I don't understand my treatments & I'm scared about side-effects

Emotional response
Anxiety
Low mood
Lack of confidence
Overwhelmed
Self-blame

Behaviour
Avoiding looking at psoriasis
Lots of dieting
Fearful of missing treatments
Hiding and avoiding
Missed opportunities

In this second example, a woman in her twenties has suffered with psoriasis since her teens but has always felt so anxious about it that she has never sought information from health professionals or the internet. She doesn't really understand what is happening to her body and she doesn't know how the treatments work and what are side effects or symptoms of psoriasis. She avoids looking at her skin and misses out on going to places. When she has a sudden flare-up, she is overwhelmed by anxiety and thinks it must be something she has done. This leads her to go on a restricted diet, but she doesn't feel confident this will work and her mood sinks.

FIGURE 10.2 Case studies illustrating how illness beliefs can drive behaviour and feelings

their control, like genetics. This led me to recognise the importance of being given clear, accurate information about the complex and multi-factorial causes of psoriasis.

These findings are interesting to me as a psychologist. They're also very important to me as someone with psoriasis because they remind me of the ways in which my beliefs about psoriasis drive my behaviour and efforts to cope. It's not often that we analyse our beliefs and thoughts or ask ourselves where they came from or question their accuracy. But they are significant, influencing how we feel about ourselves and, more importantly, determining how we act.

The benefits of self-knowledge

It can be helpful to examine your beliefs. Just think what you might do differently if you realised that deep down you believe you'll never get psoriasis under control. If you were able to identify and then challenge that belief, instead of feeling hopeless and avoiding a visit to the doctor for advice, you might decide to look for a reputable dermatologist who can help you try new treatments.

Try this

When thinking about your psoriasis, try to answer these questions:

What do you think are the main symptoms of psoriasis?
In what ways does psoriasis affect your life?
Where do you get most of your information about psoriasis from?
Does your medication or treatments cause any side-effects?
How necessary is your medication or treatment in keeping you well?
Why do you think you developed psoriasis in the first place?
Do you think anything you're doing is making your psoriasis better or worse?
How long do you think your psoriasis will last?

> How do you think your psoriasis will be in the future?
> Do you think there will ever be a cure for psoriasis and what might it be?

Having thought through your answers to these questions, it's useful to question whether your beliefs are accurate by looking for online information from trustworthy sources, like the Psoriasis Association in the UK, or talking them over at your next clinic appointment.

Once you know what your beliefs are, you can start to understand why you cope with psoriasis in the way you do. For example, I've always been reluctant to try systemic medication for my skin (drug therapies like tablets or injections that work throughout the whole body) and I know this comes from my beliefs about 'natural' cures, that I should be able to control my psoriasis by making health-conscious choices, eating the right foods, meditating and exercising. This is a good example of an implicit belief I've never put under the microscope. I also hold the belief that a systemic treatment might be dangerous for me.

Two experiences were important in forming my belief that systemic treatments should be avoided if possible. First, I remember reading about the playwright Dennis Potter at the end of his life in 1994. He'd started taking a tablet medication to manage his psoriasis and had developed terminal cancer of the liver and pancreas. I don't know if the two things were linked, but I made a connection and didn't want to risk developing terminal cancer. Now that I analyse my beliefs in more detail, I realise that I don't even know what treatment Dennis Potter was taking or whether it was linked to his cancer diagnosis. I also know that treatments have advanced considerably since the early 1990s.

The second experience happened in my late twenties at a dermatology appointment in which we discussed systemic treatment as an option. The advice of my consultant at the time was not to suppress my immune system if I could avoid it because my risk of cancer would increase. Having lost a grandmother to the disease, it was a risk I wasn't prepared to take.

I continued to hold this belief, linking systemic medication and cancer for a long time, and this put me off trying a systemic or biologic treatment. Understanding how my beliefs developed, meant I could ask for advice from my doctors and on support forums, and read the latest treatments, scientific research and evidence. This helped me to update my beliefs as new information came to light. There are good sources of information listed in the Appendix, such as the Psoriasis Association and the British Association of Dermatology, which can help you update your beliefs, and always consult your doctor before you make any changes to your treatments.

Clinicians' beliefs

The doctors who treat us are also influenced by their own beliefs. Whether or not clinicians believe psoriasis is purely a skin disease, or feel able to manage aspects of the condition other than treating the plaques, will make a huge difference to the consultation and support offered to patients. Overall, evidence suggests that clinicians and patients rate not only the severity of their psoriasis very differently but also satisfaction with treatment, with clinicians giving higher satisfaction ratings than patients who rate their satisfaction as low (Griffiths et al., 2018). This is a problem because there is a risk that treatment is based on ill-informed clinical judgements.

Clinicians' beliefs determine how they communicate with patients and whether they encourage their patients to make decisions alongside them. In one study, several medics saw their role as treating the physical symptoms only, rather than seeing psoriasis as a long-term condition with complex psychological, behavioural and social impacts (Hewitt et al., 2022). These clinicians are unlikely to enquire about mental health or limitations to daily life. More worryingly, this study found that clinicians made assumptions about patients' ability to adhere to treatment based on the patient's age and this influenced what they prescribed, limiting access to treatments for younger people.

Primary care providers (like GPs in the UK) often have limited knowledge of psoriasis with one survey estimating that the majority receive only between one and five hours of psoriasis-specific training (Kumar et al., 2021). It's not surprising then that a significant number of people with moderate-to-severe psoriasis are undertreated (Armstrong et al., 2017). Learning to manage your psoriasis alongside your care providers is crucial, and there is more information about this in Chapter 13.

Our beliefs and notions about psoriasis are crucial in determining the way we manage the condition, how we cope and the impact on our daily lives. The beliefs of our care providers can affect the care and treatments we are offered. It's therefore vital to consider your beliefs as well as learn to communicate and work with your doctor towards an informed understanding and course of treatment.

Summary

- People with psoriasis form implicit beliefs about the condition.
- These beliefs determine how they cope with it.
- Understanding your psoriasis belief system can help you correct inaccurate information and help you cope and manage better.

Top tips

- What you believe about psoriasis is really important.
- It may be hard to work out how your beliefs are affecting the way you cope.
- Start by thinking about what you think the main impact of psoriasis is.
- Next, move on to considering the beliefs questions in this chapter.
- You might find it helpful to discuss these questions and your beliefs with your doctor.
- Always consult your doctor before making any changes to your treatments.

11 Psychological strategies for coping

All humans, and not just those of us with psoriasis, have a bias towards negative thinking. It's estimated that for every positive thought we might have, there are five negative thoughts close behind.

Focusing on the negative

The existence of this bias in humans is backed up by research which shows that not only is our thinking more likely to be negative, but we pay more attention to negative experiences than positive experiences. Similarly, we're more likely to make decisions based on negative experience rather than positive experience, and by remembering and dwelling on the negative more strongly, we learn more from negative experiences than positive experiences. We have a bigger emotional and physical response to aversive stimuli than pleasant stimuli. We replay insults over and over in our heads but discount praise (Cacioppo et al., 2014). The pull towards the negative is strong.

We might get a multitude of compliments during the day, do things well and achieve our goals, but most of the time we tend to discount these successes, telling ourselves people are just being nice, or they are deluded, and that what we achieved was really no big deal. One criticism or mistake, on the other hand, will stay with us for the rest of the day, maybe even the rest of our lives. When reflecting on our day, we'll consider it a disaster because of the one thing that went wrong, forgetting all of the things that went well.

In my clinical experience, the people I work with tend to be harsh with themselves. They tell themselves off for things that go wrong, they focus on their flaws and mistakes and replay awkward and embarrassing memories over and over until they're etched on their brains. I see this in most people I meet, and not just those I see for therapy. This bias towards the negative is an unfortunate default setting in most humans.

Negativity bias and evolution

Scientists believe there is an evolutionary basis to the negativity bias (Gilbert, 2014). You may remember in Chapter 3, I wrote about our alarm system that is easily triggered in response to threat. It keeps us safe from danger by sending us into flight, fight or freeze mode when there is a danger to deal with. In order for our ancestors to protect themselves, the alarm system needed to be easily triggered by any viable threats around them. Those who responded quickly, rather than waiting around to see if it really was a dangerous situation, were much more likely to survive and pass on their genes.

Similarly, it's much more important in terms of survival to dwell on the near miss with the shark than all the fun times we swam in the sea without being attacked. The good times are not important in survival terms. Our ancestors would have needed to remember and endlessly replay near misses in order to survive and pass on their genes. The fact that in modern times we continue to dwell on negative experiences is a by-product of our evolution.

As we saw in Chapter 3, often the alarm is triggered even when the threat doesn't need action, for example when it is a memory or a worry about something that may or may not happen in the future.

Not only does this negativity bias have an impact on mental well-being, self-esteem and confidence, it's thought to be directly linked to the high rates of depression and anxiety in modern times.

Negativity bias and psoriasis

Once you understand the negativity bias, you can start to see how it can make living with psoriasis a whole lot worse. When you live with a chronic skin condition, this vulnerability to mental health struggles is magnified.

I might have had hundreds of genuine compliments about my appearance over the years, yet the negative comments, though far fewer, have stuck with me. Even well-meaning, though insensitive, comments (like 'what's wrong with your legs?' and 'that looks sore') are much more memorable. I replay them over in my mind, and they start to form strongly held beliefs about myself and my appearance. They impact my choices, where I go and how I dress. I keep discounting the compliments as they no longer fit with my body image.

This tendency towards negative thinking means that we are prone to making errors, like misperceiving how others are judging us and believing that because our psoriasis is obvious to us, it's obvious to others too.

One of my friends with psoriasis told me that she hates to sit in the cinema or theatre with people behind her because the whole time she's imagining they are looking at the psoriasis on her scalp and the flakes on her shoulders, and judging her for scratching her head all the time.

This happens to me when I wear shorts and I imagine that everyone is looking at my legs. For this reason, I'm uncomfortable when people walk behind me. I'm convinced I can mindread what others are thinking about me. The fact that I can't see their faces lets my imagination run wild with fanciful images of disgusted expressions.

Types of thinking errors

Psychologists have labelled different types of thinking errors, and you might find that you do some of these too (Figure 11.1).

These thinking errors, or cognitive distortions, if used often enough, repeatedly trigger our threat system. In the long term, this has the potential to make us feel depressed, out of control and anxious. The way we think affects not just how we feel but also what we do or don't do. This might be clearer if you consider the following example:

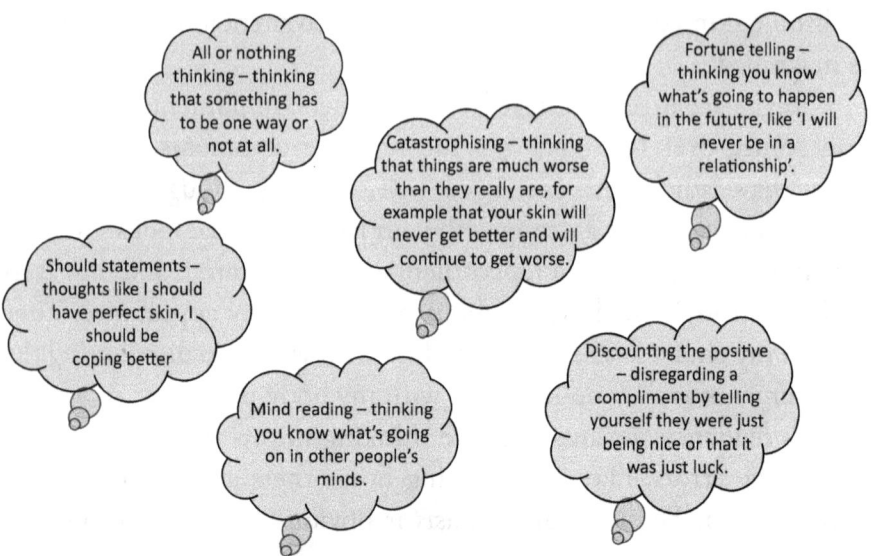

FIGURE 11.1 Types of thinking errors

Case Study

Situation A

It's the second week of July and so far, it has been a great summer. Up until this point, Rebecca has been wearing long sleeves and trousers to hide her psoriasis, but today she can't take the heat any longer and has decided to wear a skirt and T-shirt to her friend's house. As she leaves, her Mum tells her she looks nice. Rebecca tells herself her Mum is just saying that to make her feel better [Thinking error: discounting the positive].

Rebecca walks down the high street and past a group of teenagers who are hanging out on the street corner. As she passes them, they start laughing. Her mind whirrs with the following thoughts:

> *Those kids are laughing at my skin. They must think I'm disgusting.* [Thinking error: mind reading].

It looks hideous. [Thinking error: catastrophising].

I should have worn trousers and long sleeves. [Thinking error: should].

What's the point? I'll never be able to lead a normal life. [Thinking error: fortune telling].

Rebecca blushes and feels hot and embarrassed. She turns down the next street and instead of going to her friend's house, she walks home fighting back tears. When she gets there, she changes into trousers.

Situation B

It's the second week of July and so far, it has been a great summer. Up until this point, Rebecca has been wearing long sleeves and trousers to hide her psoriasis, but today she can't take the heat any longer and has decided to wear a skirt and T-shirt to her friend's house. As she leaves, her Mum tells her she looks nice and Rebecca looks down at her new top which she loves and smiles.

Rebecca walks down the high street and past a group of teenagers who are hanging out on the street corner. As she passes them, they start laughing. This prompts her to think, 'Teenagers seem to find everything so funny. I wonder what they are laughing about. I bet they are talking about boys. I can remember being like that'. Rebecca starts to daydream and remember happy times from her youth. She arrives at her friend's house feeling happy.

Situation C

It's the second week of July and so far, it has been a great summer. Up until this point, Rebecca has been wearing long sleeves and trousers to hide her psoriasis, but today she can't take the heat any longer and has decided to wear a skirt and T-shirt to her friend's house. As she leaves, her Mum tells her she looks nice. Rebecca knows her Mum always tells the truth and she thanks her for the

> compliment. Even though she thinks her legs look sore, she likes the outfit she's chosen, and she's pleased with her new haircut.
>
> Rebecca walks down the high street and past a group of teenagers who are hanging out on the street corner. As she passes them, they start laughing. Her first thought is, 'I wonder if they are laughing at me'. But then she tells herself, 'I doubt it. I don't suppose they noticed me at all and anyway, psoriasis isn't that funny'. She listens to some music for the rest of the journey, forgetting all about the teenagers. She arrives at her friend's house feeling relaxed.

In each of these examples, it's exactly the same situation, but because the *thoughts* are different, the consequent feelings and behaviour are quite different too. Who knows what the teenagers were laughing at? They might have found the sight of Rebecca's arms and legs hilarious. They might not have. Rebecca will never know, but what she thought about the situation had a big impact on the way she felt about herself and how she experienced the rest of her day.

Cognitive Behavioural Therapy

The idea that we have a tendency towards negative information, and we make thinking errors but believe and act on our thoughts as if they were the truth, forms the basis of Cognitive Behavioural Therapy (CBT). It's an effective therapy which helps people start to become more aware of their thought processes and then challenge unhelpful thinking.

Had Rebecca in Situation A applied a CBT approach, she would have noticed she was feeling distressed and then made a note of what she had been thinking and what thinking errors she'd made. She would then challenge her thoughts with more helpful alternatives (like the examples given in Situations B and C). Over time, awareness of thinking errors and the ability to challenge them becomes second nature.

We know from research that CBT can improve depression and anxiety, and a review of five trials of CBT as a treatment for psoriasis also found improvements in the severity of psoriasis (Xiao et al., 2019).

If you are interested in finding out more about CBT, there are excellent sources of information online, including the British Association for Behavioural and Cognitive Psychotherapies.

Acceptance and Commitment Therapy

In my clinical practice, I'm more likely to use Acceptance and Commitment Therapy (ACT), a form of CBT that has proved especially useful for people living with chronic health conditions. ACT works on the same basic principles as CBT, that our thinking can be overly negative and unhelpful and can affect the way we feel and what we do.

ACT differs slightly from CBT in that it teaches people to notice thoughts for what they are: not truths but fallible perceptions. Instead of getting into a battle about the correctness of your thinking and challenging or changing thoughts, in ACT you simply put your thoughts to one side and instead focus on what's important to you.

For example, say my children want me to take them to the beach for the day. There's a chance we'll run into people we know, which makes me worry. I love spending time at the beach but my immediate thought will be whether I can wear a swimming costume and risk exposing my psoriasis, and I worry how people will judge me if they see my skin. I imagine the shame I might feel if we bump into someone we know.

Using an ACT approach, I notice the negative direction my thoughts have taken and how one negative thought is leading to another in quick succession. I recognise that I'm starting to catastrophise and fortune tell, imagining I'll bump into people from work and neighbours and everyone will be shocked and disgusted at the sight of my legs.

Using a CBT approach, I would spot my thinking errors and challenge my thoughts by replacing them with more helpful ones. With ACT, instead of getting caught up in this train of thoughts, I say to myself, 'There I go telling myself the story where everyone notices my skin and is disgusted by it'. Just that simple trick of noticing that what is going through my head is simply my thoughts and not the truth allows me to take a step back.

We call the stepping back from thoughts cognitive defusion because it allows us to be less 'fused' with our thinking and believing our thoughts reflect reality accurately. In ACT, there is an acceptance that as humans we'll have negative thoughts and feelings and from time to time we'll feel pain and discomfort, and that's just a part of life. The acceptance part refers to the method of not resisting or struggling against negative thoughts or unpleasant feelings but instead accepting them.

Passengers on a bus: a visual metaphor for ACT

Many ACT therapists use the metaphor of passengers on a bus, originally created by psychologist Dr Steven Hayes (Hayes et al., 2016), to explain how ACT works.

Imagine you're a bus driver and you have a destination you want to get to. Unfortunately, your bus is full of really unpleasant passengers. They're shouting at you and telling you that you're a terrible bus driver and you're never going to get to your destination and that they don't want to go where you're heading.

For a while, you stop the bus, put the handbrake on and argue back with them. You end up feeling exhausted. Then, you try and make deals with them and drive them where they want to go. They're a bit quieter, but now you're not heading to your preferred destination (Figure 11.2).

You eventually stop the bus and try to get the passengers off, but they refuse to leave, and now the bus is not moving at all (Figure 11.3).

The passengers don't touch you or physically hurt you, and they're not taking control of the steering wheel, but they intimidate you and you can't concentrate on the route. As a consequence, you take wrong turns and end up driving around in circles. All the while, you're feeling miserable and the passengers are never satisfied.

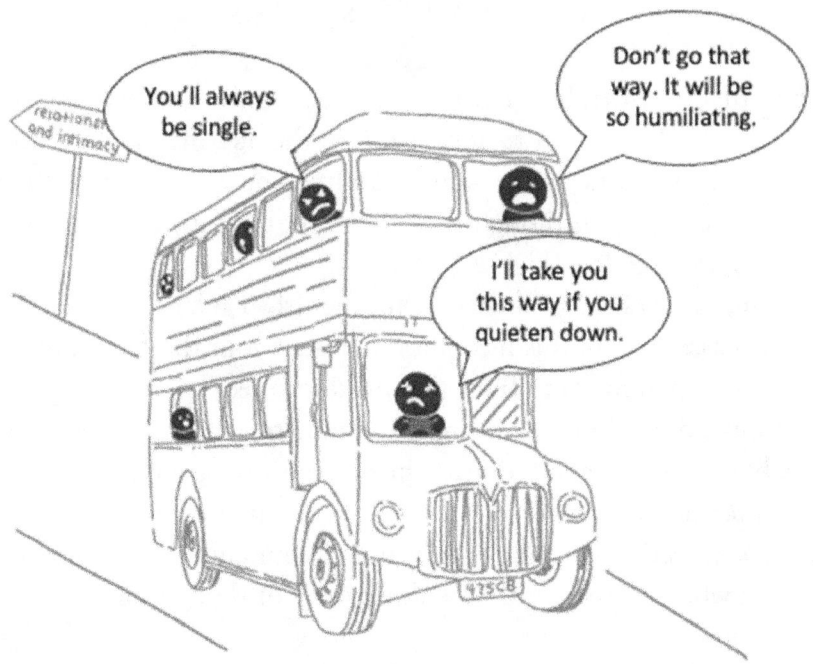

FIGURE 11.2 The defeated bus driver

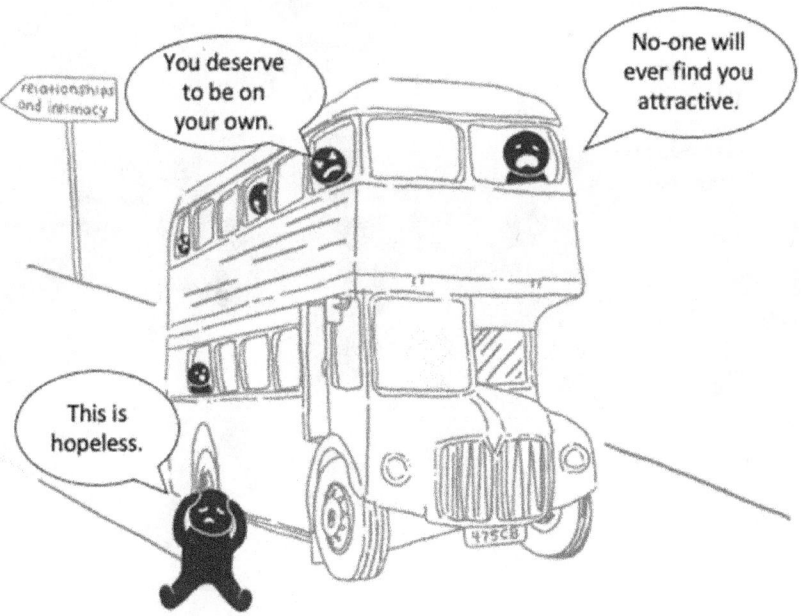

FIGURE 11.3 The despairing bus driver

Eventually you realise that the passengers only have the power to intimidate and since they're not getting off the bus, instead you choose to let them moan in the background while you concentrate on your route. This way, even though they're still on the bus, you're going in your chosen direction (Figure 11.4).

Having psoriasis is a bit like being the driver of the Psoriasis Bus, and the passengers in this metaphor represent your thoughts and feelings. They're telling you things that make you feel miserable and stop you from doing things that are important to you. Like me, you've probably tried either fighting them or even giving in to them, but when that happens, you start to take your bus in the wrong direction. The direction your life takes is not of your choosing. You need to focus on where you want to go and not on your thoughts and feelings, which run their own course.

This is a different strategy to simply ignore unpleasant thoughts and feelings, nor is it pretending to yourself that things are fine. In ACT, you notice your difficult thoughts and feelings, acknowledge them and

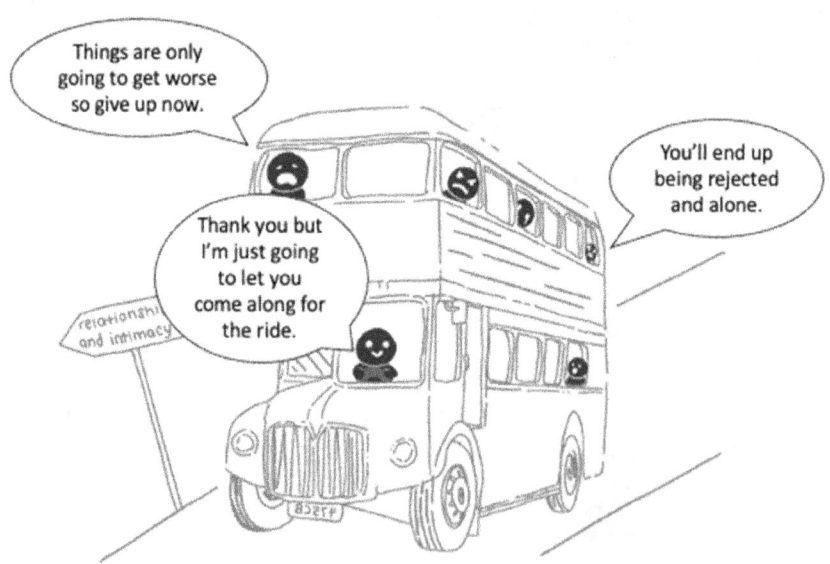

FIGURE 11.4 The ACT bus driver

then choose to focus your attention on something that brings your life value and meaning. You let the passengers join you for the ride regardless of what they're telling you.

Letting go of the struggle

Struggling against unpleasant thoughts and feelings means that all our focus and energy are directed at the struggle and there's no room for anything else in our lives. Your life becomes all about the negative thoughts and the unpleasant feelings they bring along with them. Has it ever felt to you that your battle with psoriasis is all consuming? In ACT, we're encouraged to let go of the struggle. I wrote about this in Chapter 7, where I described letting go of the rope in tug of war against pain.

It can help to check in with yourself and notice your thinking, especially if it seems that your thoughts are racing, stuck in the same old groove or repeating over and over. At times when you're caught up in your thinking and not paying attention to the outside world, you might need to do some defusion. Notice the story you're telling yourself. Give it a label like, 'This is the story where I tell myself I'll never succeed because I have psoriasis'. Remind yourself that your thoughts are just thoughts.

Taking action

The other important part of ACT is the commitment to take action and make positive changes in your life. We do this by considering what our values are and what's important to us. This is the destination you're heading to on your bus.

It's important to set aside some time to do this exercise properly. Consider the following questions:

What's important to you?
What sort of person do you want to be?
What do you want to be remembered for?

This is not always easy. First, we often get muddled between – on the one hand – material things (like a new car) and goals (like getting a high grade in your exams) and – on the other hand – values (the qualities that are important to us). For example, a goal is something concrete that's achievable, like getting a promotion at work, whereas a value is more about striving in a particular direction you want your life to go in, like being creative, wise, useful or courageous.

If you continue to struggle with thinking about your values, then you could try the following exercise.

> **Try this**
>
> **Values exercise**
>
> Imagine it's your 80th birthday and one by one all the important people in your life say something about you and what you meant to them.
>
> What do you hope you'll hear?
> Write these valued qualities down. They're the important ones.

Think about all the time you spend doing things that don't move you in a direction consistent with your values. Instead, what are the things you could be doing that would help you feel more fulfilled in life?

My values include being caring, compassionate, hard-working, reliable and fun. These are the values I need to focus on in work and in my home life. My committed actions, even when my psoriasis is bad and I'm feeling overwhelmed, would include spending time with my family and taking opportunities for fun that come my way. I need to make sure at work that my actions and goals are in line with my values too.

Living in the present

The final part of ACT is learning to live in the present moment. All too easily our thinking can drag us back into the past or project us into the future. Because of the negativity bias, it's likely that our minds will take us to unpleasant memories and frightening futures; all the while, we miss paying attention to the present. I find mindfulness a really useful strategy to help me be in the present.

I was working at Guy's Hospital in London when I did my first training in ACT. As part of the course, we were instructed to walk around the outside of the hospital mindfully. It was a route I'd done countless times on my daily commute. Most often I rushed from the tube station to the hospital building on autopilot with my mind focused on the day ahead and the tasks I needed to fulfil.

This time, however, we were invited to walk slowly, noticing our footfall on the floor beneath us. We were asked to look at the buildings, to notice the plants. We felt the temperature and observed the sounds and smells of a busy London thoroughfare. We were asked to walk slower than we normally would and experience walking as a sensation alongside our breath, our balance and the movement of our limbs. It was like nothing I'd ever done before. For the first time in my years of working at Guy's, I noticed the brickwork and the gardens, even the weeds poking up from the tarmac, and I appreciated the way my body moved me forward.

I was not trying to get anywhere. I was simply walking. Until I looked up and spotted the whole group of us doing the same thing and the perplexed looks of passers-by, and I got uncontrollable giggles. It's not unusual for someone to find it amusing when I'm teaching mindfulness, and that always makes me laugh too. As I've become more practised in mindfulness, I know giggling is allowed and a wandering mind is normal. Both will happen. The important thing is just to notice what's happened and carry on.

I often try to walk mindfully now, especially with my dog. She's not fretting over getting muddy yesterday or criticising herself for barking so aggressively at the sweet little dog on the corner. She's not worrying about whether she'll be given a bath later, though she hates them and she needs one. She's just in the moment, enjoying my company, the sights and mainly the smells of the present. Why not try mindful walking yourself, with or without a dog?

Promoting quality of life through ACT

There's good evidence that ACT can help people with chronic illness to have a better quality of life. In 2019, a clinical psychologist called Dr Jo Tedstone recorded a powerful video chronicling how ACT had helped her make the most of the end of her life following a diagnosis of terminal cancer. It's a very moving account of the way she copes with her diagnosis and a good example of how ACT, which she'd been using in her clinical work, can help. Dr Tedstone's family was also struggling and she explained it to them in the following way:

> Yes, I am dying ... these difficult thoughts and emotions are going to crop up, you don't squash them away and pretend they're not there. You acknowledge that they're there but in quite a brief way. So yes, I'm noticing that I'm worrying about what that new pain there might be, make space for it, open up around it and then become present again and do something that you value and engage in life again in the present.

There's emerging evidence that people with psoriasis tend to be fused with their thinking about their body image, telling themselves that just because they think something about the way they look it is the truth (Almeida et al., 2020). By engaging in ACT (cognitive defusion, committed action and living in the present), people with psoriasis can feel better about themselves (Zucchelli et al., 2022).

Over the past 10 chapters, we've learnt a lot about the experience of living with psoriasis and psoriatic arthritis (PsA). The symptoms and treatments sap our energy and limit what we can physically do. Our feelings of shame and low self-esteem lead us to hide and avoid situations. Past experiences have left us feeling stigmatised and traumatised. We might shut down emotionally in order to cope. We might start drinking and eating junk food as a comfort or conversely diet and restrict what we think might be 'bad' foods. We begin to mindread and assume others are judging us negatively and we dwell on the times someone commented on our skin. All this impacts on how we relate to other people and to ourselves.

It might seem that we're victims of our evolution and that we've inherited minds that were built to ensure our ancestors' survival, but ACT can help us do something about it. It takes deliberate effort to correct our negative bias, but knowing and understanding it is the first step in learning how to manage it. This can be achieved through mindful acceptance and leading a life true to our values. The next chapter will explore ways to develop self-compassion and other strategies to change the attentional bias in a more positive direction.

Summary

- Our minds have evolved to protect us, but that means we pay more attention to negative information.
- Life is like driving a bus and your bus will have unruly passengers on it, which are our thoughts and feelings.
- Your thoughts are simply thoughts. Just because you think something, doesn't make it true.
- Work out what your values for life are and take committed action to live accordingly.
- Live in the present, not as a prisoner of the past or a hostage to the future.

Top tips

- Try to notice when your attention and thinking is drawn to the negative.
- Instead of dismissing a compliment, listen and take it on board.
- It can help to keep a diary and write down what happened during the day and what was going through your mind. See if you can spot any thinking errors.
- Remind yourself that your thoughts are just thoughts.
- Practise mindfulness to help you live in the present.

12 Developing self-compassion

If you want others to be happy, practice compassion. If you want to be happy, practice compassion.

— Dalai Lama

I consider the single most important thing you can do when you have psoriasis is to be kind and compassionate to yourself, in exactly the same way you would show compassion for someone you love.

Self-compassion and self-kindness is not a skill that comes naturally or instinctively to most people. Countering the feelings of shame, low mood and frustration with understanding and self-caring might seem obvious, but for most people, it's a completely novel approach. Even people with strong compassion for others find it hard to regard themselves with the same level of kindness. Instead, we find it easy to speak to ourselves in very harsh and critical ways, telling ourselves we look awful and that we're failing, which makes us feel ashamed and unworthy.

Understanding the importance of self-compassion

To understand the importance of self-compassion for well-being and coping with psoriasis, try the following exercise. Our self-critical voices are often so entrenched, it can be easier to understand the logic behind it if you're thinking about someone you care about.

Try this

Developing self-compassion exercise

Imagine your best friend or close relative contacts you and asks for your help. They are working away from home and something has cropped up that means they're not going to make it home tonight as planned. They have an appointment at the gym to choose a personal trainer, and as there's a waiting list for these appointments, they don't want to miss it. They ask if you can go instead. You know how much this means to them. They're starting to make changes in life, which includes getting fit, and so you're happy to help.

When you get to the gym, the manager tells you that two personal trainers are available so you can meet them both and decide. The first trainer greets you enthusiastically. Let's call her Agnes.

Agnes is working with a client and sets them up to do sit-ups while she turns to talk to you. She tells you she wants the best for her clients, and that she'll work hard to help your friend reach their full potential. With that, the client who has been doing sit-ups groans loudly and lies flat out. Immediately, Agnes turns and barks at the client in a harsh tone, 'Why have you stopped? Keep going. You need to do 20 reps. This is pathetic. You're pathetic. You can't have done more than five. Everyone is looking at you. You're never going to get rid of that flabby belly. You've got no stamina. Other people would have found this workout easy. Just lie there and think about how pathetic you're being'.

Agnes turns back to you and tells you that she never settles for less than the best and she thinks the only way to motivate someone is to point out their flaws and respond quickly to weakness with harsh criticism. Agnes tells you she thinks people learn best when they are strongly motivated to change.

You go on to meet the second trainer, Jenny. She also has a client she's working with at that moment, and she leaves them doing push-ups while she talks to you. Jenny tells you that she wants all her clients to achieve their full potential, and she works hard to help people achieve their best.

With that, there's a moan and her client stops doing push-ups and lies face down on the mat. Jenny goes over to them and asks if they're alright. The client tells her they can't do any more. Jenny says, 'Okay. You've done two sets of push-ups today. Maybe you need a rest and then we can try a few more. You're doing really great and I can see the difference you're making. Remember how you couldn't even manage one set when you started? You've exceeded that today. Take five minutes and we'll have a rethink of today's plan, see if we can do another set, and then maybe spend the rest of this session on leg exercises'.

Jenny then comes back to you and says, 'I feel people develop best when the coaching is thoughtful and encouraging. It helps when people recognise their achievements and see the changes they're making'.

When you go back to the manager, which trainer would you choose: Agnes or Jenny?
Which trainer is more likely to help your friend or loved one succeed?
Which trainer will keep them more motivated?
Which one is likely to help them get fit?

I'm guessing, like me, you would pick the second one. If you've seen the 2014 film *Whiplash*, or read Roald Dahl's *Matilda*, you'll know that the style of teaching based on criticism, fear and intimidation rarely works in the long term. If your friend or relative had a trainer who belittled them and judged them harshly, they would start to feel miserable at the gym. It might even cause them to make mistakes. If they were constantly told they were useless and failing, and any successes were dismissed, they would probably give up entirely.

Psoriasis and the self-critical voice

For many people with psoriasis, when they look in the mirror, eat badly or forget to use their treatments, or make mistakes in other areas of their lives, they talk to themselves in exactly the same manner as Agnes the trainer addresses the people she coaches at the gym. They tell themselves they look disgusting and ugly, that they're useless and not doing anything to alleviate the condition.

This doesn't help people to manage their psoriasis better, nor is there any greater likelihood that their psoriasis will improve if they're critical of themselves. It just makes someone feel low and miserable.

We wouldn't talk to someone we loved in the same way, and it's easy to see why. We'd tell them about how great we thought they were, how much we admired their courage, how we were there for them, to support them. We would be gentle and supportive and help them to keep going when times were tough. That's just the kind of thing we need to learn to say to ourselves.

Our inner voice and emotional regulation

The way we speak to ourselves determines how our emotions are regulated. Psychologists believe we have three systems regulating our emotions: threat, drive and soothe (Gilbert, 2010). At any one time, we are in one of these systems. They're all essential for our survival, but when they are out of balance, you can end up feeling exhausted, overwhelmed and distressed.

When our inner voice talks to us with kindness and compassion, we are more likely to feel calm and cared for. In contrast, when our inner voice is critical and unkind, we're likely to feel under threat or driven to resolve something. Both of these emotional states take us away from doing activities that are soothing and essential for our mental and physical well-being.

A critical inner voice will activate your **THREAT** system, and it can help to think of this as your alarm that goes off when you're in a dangerous situation. Working on a 'better safe than sorry approach', for most people it's a very sensitive system triggered by even slight threats.

When we're in threat mode, our heart rate and blood pressure are raised, and our bodies get flooded with stress hormones like adrenaline and cortisol. Our body prepares itself to fight, run away from danger or freeze. External dangers, like a fire, could activate the threat system, and that would help us to react and stay safe. Importantly, our thinking and self-critical thoughts can also trigger the threat response. So we might end up in threat mode when we remember something from the past, worry about something that may happen in the future or tell ourselves that we look disgusting and that people won't want to be around us.

Thoughts like 'you should be doing more to get rid of your psoriasis' and 'this is all your fault for eating the wrong thing and not losing weight' are likely to activate our **DRIVE** system. It's an important system because it spurs us to take action. It's what helps us feel motivated and gets us out of bed in the morning to get things done. Our drive system pushes us to strive for things, like doing well at work or training for a big event like a marathon.

When we're in drive mode, we get a rush of a brain chemical called dopamine, which gives us a buzz. Our thinking narrows, there are changes in our sleep and we're very focused on achievement. If your drive system is activated all the time, you'd end up feeling burnt out. I experience drive mode through my thoughts that I'm eating the wrong thing or not trying hard enough to manage my psoriasis, sending me searching for new diet and exercise plans. This might be helpful in the short-term but you can see how it can become overwhelming and exhausting over time.

A critical inner voice never activates the **SOOTHE** system, our caregiving mode. When we feel cared for, we get a surge of a brain chemical called oxytocin, sometimes called the love hormone. We feel calm, relaxed and kinder towards ourselves. Everything is much slower and we can recharge our batteries.

Balancing threat, drive and soothe systems

When you have psoriasis, there's a lot that can push you into threat mode in addition to a self-critical inner voice – for example, a flare-up, a hospital appointment, leaving flakes of skin at your work desk, feeling judged and ashamed, fearing that it's out of control and so on.

There are also many possible triggers to put you into drive mode, like using your treatments correctly, trying the next recommended diet or alternative therapy, feeling you've got to overhaul your lifestyle, vacuuming constantly to rid your home of skin flakes, going to great lengths to hide away your skin in different ways, etc (Figure 12.1).

This means we can spend all our time bouncing between feeling under threat and driven to take action, with little or no opportunity to activate our soothe system. We don't do the things that make us

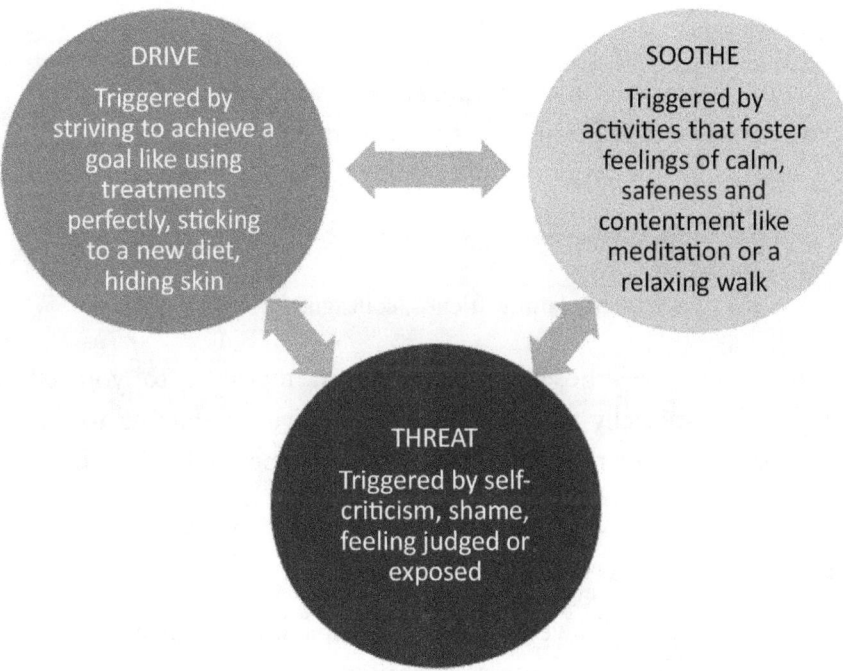

FIGURE 12.1 How psoriasis can impact the emotional regulation system. Source: Adapted from Gilbert, 2010

feel calm, content and cared for. It's not surprising we often feel overwhelmed and worn-out by our experience of psoriasis.

The power of self-affirmation

The good news is that there are things you can do to quieten your self-critical voice and develop your more compassionate voice. One study has looked at the impact of using self-affirmation in psoriasis (Łakuta, 2021). People were asked to use positive sentiments, like thinking about the things they value in themselves, at times when they felt low or anxious, over a two-week period. The results showed that self-affirmation resulted in reduced depression and anxiety and increased feelings of well-being. There were also trends towards fewer negative feelings about their body and appearance.

> **Try this**
>
> To put this technique into action at times when you feel distressed, you can choose affirmations of your own such as:
>
> > 'I am loved'.
> > 'I am not defined by psoriasis'.
> > 'I am worthy'.
> > 'I am valued by my family, friends, colleagues'.
>
> Once you have chosen an affirmation, repeat it to yourself regularly, especially when you notice that you're starting to feel low or anxious or that your thinking has become self-critical.

Activating your soothe system

An important part of developing your compassionate voice and caring for yourself is learning how to activate your soothe system. Many people spend so much time bouncing between threat and drive, that they've forgotten what helps them to feel soothed.

Developing self-compassion

Activities that activate my soothe system include walking my dog on the beach, curling up with a hot drink and a good book, using aromatherapy and taking a moment to meditate.

Sometimes, it can feel like these types of activities are self-indulgent or a low priority, but that's not the case. Without soothing activities, things can quickly feel out of balance, and people tend not to function well in any aspect of their lives.

You may wish to try a self-compassion meditation to help you channel feelings of calm and contentment. You can listen to an audio version of this script at: www.copingwithpsoriasis.com.

Try this

Self-compassion meditation

Start this exercise by getting yourself comfortable. You can lie down or sit in a chair if you prefer, but try not to have any outside distractions, so turn off the television or radio and allow yourself ten minutes to meditate undisturbed.

Start by becoming aware of your breath. There's no need to change how you're breathing, don't alter the speed or depth of each breath. Instead, just notice your breathing. Follow each breath as it comes in through your mouth or nose, down into your lungs and then follow it out of your body again, without trying to change it. Just be aware of each breath as it comes into and out of your body.

Throughout this exercise, if any distracting thoughts arise, just notice them. Don't get involved but instead return to focusing on your breath.

In this meditation, we'll begin to develop compassion for ourselves. This can feel hard, so we'll start by thinking about someone who you feel warmth and affection towards. Think about a person in your life who you feel happy to see and to whom you feel affection. It might be someone from your past or a child you care for. It might even be a beloved pet. Take a moment to really bring them to mind and notice the feelings that arise when you think of them. You may feel a sense of warmth or tenderness. You may feel like smiling. As you bring that person or pet to mind, allow all the feelings and sensations to arise in your body. Stay with them for a few moments.

> Think of that person and send them thoughts of love and compassion. Send them good wishes and thoughts of kindness and love. In your mind, say: 'I wish you peace and contentment'.
> 'May you feel at ease'.
> 'May you feel calm and relaxed'.

Stay with those feelings for a while. Now while still holding those feelings of warmth and compassion in mind, turn your attention to yourself. See if you can find the same feelings of compassion and kindness for yourself. Allow yourself to send those same feelings of tenderness to yourself. In your mind, say to yourself:

> 'May I be contented'.
> 'May I live in peace, no matter what I face'.
> 'May I be calm and relaxed'.
> 'May I feel at ease despite psoriasis'

Notice the feelings and sensations that arise and let them be.

Sit with them for a few moments until you are ready to end the exercise.

If this resonated with you, you may wish to try a loving-kindness meditation which is an extended version of this meditation. It's one I often practice, and always find to be especially soothing and calming. It gives me a real sense of compassion and warmth for others that then extends to having the same feelings towards myself. It improves my well-being and I urge you to try it. There's evidence that meditations focused on compassion and loving-kindness not only improve psychological well-being, but neuroendocrine studies show that they can reduce stress and induced distress and immune response to stress (Hofmann et al., 2011). There are many recorded versions available online and you could try a few until you settle on a voice and script you like.

Other self-compassion techniques

There are other things you can do to develop more self-compassion. Try these exercises adapted from Kirsten Neff's self-compassion website (see the resources section in the Appendix for more details):

Being your own best friend

1. Think about someone you know who is struggling right now. They might have a health condition, maybe even psoriasis, or they may be going through a difficult time at work or in their relationships. Think about how they must be feeling and how you want them to feel instead. Write down what you would say to them to let them know they're not alone, that you're there to support them and that things will get easier to manage.
2. Now reflect on the last time you felt bad about your skin. Was it in a changing room, in a shop with the mirrors reflecting your appearance from every angle? Was it after your shower? Was it during your last hair appointment? Write down what you said to yourself.
3. Now put those two lists side by side and look at the differences.
4. Imagine yourself back in that scenario, and instead of what you actually said to yourself, say the things you would have said to your friend, rewording them so the context fits for you. Write them down.
5. Finally, read the third list through. How does that make you feel? Would it make a difference if you could respond to yourself that

way at times when you're struggling? The psoriasis would still be there, but would you feel differently about yourself?
6. The next time you're bombarded with self-critical thoughts, ask yourself: How would I treat my best friend? What can I say to myself that I would tell my best friend?

Soothing touch

1. Cross your arms in front of you and rub the tops of your arms with the opposite hand using a gentle and soothing touch. This is the kind of touch we would offer a child who had hurt themselves or someone we cared about who was crying.
2. Do this for a minute or longer if it feels appropriate. Allow yourself to feel comforted and soothed by the touch.
3. Some people like to place a hand on their heart, on their chest or on the side of their face. Experiment and see what feels most soothing for you.
4. You may have patches of psoriasis on the skin you're touching. Try to touch them without judgement and instead focus your attention on the comforting feeling.

Writing yourself a compassionate letter

1. This exercise might take a little longer. Focus on your younger self and write a letter that would have helped you at that time. Don't worry about grammar or spelling. The important thing is to write something meaningful to you.
2. Think about your struggles at that time and how that made you feel. Write it down. Knowing that people with psoriasis often push down their emotions, this might feel tricky, but stick with it.
3. Write to your younger self with understanding, loving-kindness and compassion. Focus on the difficulties and what you needed to hear to help you cope with them. This isn't the time for telling your younger self to have courage or just get on with it. Instead,

acknowledge how difficult things are and how remarkable you are to keep going. Remind yourself of all the great things about your younger self.
4. Put the letter to one side. At a later time or day, come back to it and read it aloud carefully. Focus on how it makes you feel. I expect some sadness for your younger self but also a feeling of being cared for.
5. If you want an example, there is a letter in Appendix, which I wrote once during Psoriasis Awareness week. I wish I could have read it when I was younger. Reading it now helps me feel compassion and kindness towards my current self and my ongoing struggle with psoriasis.

Growing self-awareness

Now that you've read this chapter, I hope you'll become more aware of your self-critical voice and notice the times when you use it.

Even though being compassionate to yourself makes perfect common sense, it's not always easy to do. Recently, a client who was very self-critical was pleased to tell me she'd noticed her self-critical voice during a meeting at work and told herself, 'why are you being so silly again? Why do you keep doing this?'. In effect, using a self-critical voice to criticise herself for being self-critical. A more compassionate response might have included reminding herself how ingrained these habits are and how she was doing a good job of noticing her self-critical voice.

As an entrenched habit, self-critical commentary isn't always easy to spot, but that doesn't mean the habit can't be broken. Sometimes people feel nervous about quieting their critical voice in case it leads them to failure or they become conceited and big-headed. But you have to remind yourself of the Personal Trainers, Agnes and Jenny, in the exercise at the start of this chapter, and how a critical voice is unlikely to lead to long-term success and well-being. It takes lots of practise to respond to yourself with kindness. Noticing the self-critical voice and responding with a kind, compassionate voice is the first step.

I hope as you read through this book, you have started to become more aware of your internal world, your thinking patterns and feelings and how these drive behaviour and decision-making.

You can recognise that your skin might have got worse and it might look and feel sore, but instead of telling yourself that you're disgusting or a failure, remind yourself we are all imperfect beings but living with psoriasis is hard and there are things to feel good about. Recognise that feeling inadequate is part of being human. It's something everyone feels at one time or another. Countering those feelings with kindness and compassion can help you to cope better.

Summary

- Most of us talk to ourselves with a self-critical inner voice.
- Being self-critical can lead to feelings of threat and drive and can make us feel overwhelmed and exhausted.
- Self-compassion can help you feel better psychologically and physically.
- Self-compassion doesn't come easily to many of us.
- There are exercises you can do to help develop self-compassion.
- It may take time and effort, but it is possible to start treating yourself with more kindness and care.

Top tips

- Self-criticism won't help you achieve your goals or feel better.
- If things go badly, try responding to yourself with kindness and compassion.
- It can help to ask yourself how you would talk to a loved one in the same situation.
- Make sure you're doing things during the day that help you feel calm, content and cared for.

13 Coping with treatments

Since childhood, I'd always managed my psoriasis with ointments and phototherapy, and tried different diets and alternative treatments, interspersed with sunny holidays. Then, at a recent dermatology appointment, I was fully geared up to start systemic treatment.

At the previous appointment, I'd cried and explained how fed up I was with the constant struggle. I told my dermatologist that even after phototherapy, when the skin on my body was clear, I still had itchy, flaky skin all over my scalp. I couldn't remember a time when my ears didn't itch, and I felt self-conscious about tying my hair back. I was tired of planning my life around my skin, worrying about flare-ups and what clothes I would be able to wear to social or work events long before they came around.

We talked about my options for treatment. For months I'd been on the waiting list to start phototherapy, and I was wondering how practical it was to start again given how time-consuming the appointments would be. The doctor, whom I'd never met before, suggested I could try a systemic treatment, explaining there could be side effects but that many people found relief without too many problems. I asked about biologic treatments, having read about success stories on support forums, and the doctor explained they would prefer to start with a tried and tested systemic treatment, moving on to a newer biologic treatment if that option failed.

The dermatologist suggested beginning the systemic treatment with methotrexate, an immunosuppressant medication designed to reduce the body's immune response and inflammation. The biologic treatments instead target specific parts of the immune system, rather than the entire immune system, and whilst studies are showing good treatment outcomes, my dermatologist felt it would be sensible to first try a treatment with many years of research behind it. I agreed to the plan and was sent away with forms for my bloods to be checked and one for a baseline chest X-ray; all routine procedures before starting a systemic treatment.

I felt resigned but hopeful. I've worked with patients post lung and kidney transplants for many years and it gave me confidence to know so many people who coped well with these types of medications. Though I was confident another course of phototherapy would do the trick in the short term, I was drained by the constant cycle of treatments, not to mention the challenge of attending an outpatient appointment three times a week for up to three months. In contrast, the thought of managing the psoriasis by simply swallowing a tablet was very appealing.

At the following appointment, I fully expected to leave with a prescription for my first dose. This time, however, I saw a different dermatologist, one who has looked after me for several years. He advised me to stick to a course of phototherapy (by now a slot had become available) and hold off with the systemic treatments if I could.

The emotional toll of weighing treatment options

Overwhelmed by the change in plan, and partly because I'd convinced myself that methotrexate was going to work, I became emotional again, explaining how I'd had over thirty years of phototherapy followed by worsening skin and further rounds of treatment and I'd had enough.

The dermatologist's advice was to read more about the systemic treatments on offer, including one I hadn't previously considered, and to start phototherapy that week, with a follow-up appointment in a few weeks' time to discuss it further. I explained that I wanted to take a tablet and to be clear of psoriasis for the first time since I was a child. The doctor looked at me gently and reminded me there is no cure for psoriasis and all treatments have risks, so I had to make sure I was making the right decision.

Managing feelings of hopelessness

I left that appointment with a hollow feeling of hopelessness. As I walked back to my car, I had an overwhelming urge to surrender to the psoriasis. I wanted to give up, cancel all my appointments, stop putting on the creams, eat whatever I liked and just let it do its worst. That feeling of wanting to give in is something that overwhelms me from time to time.

Sergio Del Molino (del Molino Sergio, 2021) described feeling similarly after he was prescribed methotrexate, a drug he was reluctant to take after the distress of witnessing his young son take intravenous methotrexate infusions to treat leukaemia. Like me, he'd had enough of the treatments and told himself he could cope with the plaques and the aesthetic inconvenience, and he wouldn't let it interfere with his life. He just stopped all treatments. Then things took a turn for the worse and psoriasis spread across his body and affected his joints:

> *The illness has defeated me. It has surged across my body as never before [...] The discomfort has become acute and persistent, a chronic aggravation [...] There are days when no posture I assume will alleviate the pain.*

Eventually, Del Molino sought help. My own urge to surrender lasted only a few days, and after several weeks and phototherapy sessions, I was able to reflect on these very natural feelings of hopelessness.

Treatments, at best, keep psoriasis at bay. As my dermatologist reminded me, there is no cure for psoriasis. Psoriasis treatments are so different from a course of medication for an acute illness, like a viral infection, where the expected outcome is a cure. With a psoriasis treatment, you are never done. You never finish the cream when you reach the bottom of the tube because there's always the next tube lying in wait. Psoriasis treatment involves a lot of time, work and effort and often yields pretty poor results.

When you feel out of control, it's not surprising that you want to throw your arms up and give up from time to time. Although this is an understandable reaction, it may be linked to clinical depression. Look at the list of symptoms of depression in Chapter 2 and seek help if you think you might be depressed. There is a list of support and resources at the end of this book that might be of help.

Accepting the patient role

At times when you're feeling the situation is hopeless and your motivation for doing treatments is especially low, there are other ways of dealing with it rather than going cold turkey and stopping your treatment, which is likely to have detrimental effects on your health just as Del Molino discovered.

Living with psoriasis means accepting the patient role and coming to terms with the routines and treatments that go alongside the condition. Many people are lucky enough to find a treatment that works well for them, but they still need to keep doing it in order to keep symptoms at bay, maintaining regular contact with their medical team and attending appointments.

Being a patient can be a difficult role. I've spent my working life in medical settings, which adds up to decades spent in hospitals, in clinics and on wards. I'm used to working alongside doctors, nurses, pharmacists and physiotherapists. It's an environment in which I feel at ease. Yet, at times, I find being a patient challenging, and I worry about consultations, about the results of tests, about my access to treatments and about being heard and understood.

With all the focus on my condition, I often feel emotional and surprise myself by bursting into tears when answering a routine question at an appointment. It's also something I observe in the patients I see in my professional role who are similarly surprised by their emotional reaction to a routine clinic appointment.

Preparing for consultations

Part of this is a normal reaction. Emotions can feel powerful but they're not dangerous, and it's okay to cry. However, in order to get the best from every consultation, there are a few things patients can do to help prepare.

> ### Try this
>
> A good way to prepare for a clinic appointment or consultation is to consider the following questions before every appointment where new or existing treatments are discussed:
>
> 'What do I want to get out of this?'
> 'What's important to me right now?'
> 'What are my options?'
> 'What are the risks and how likely are they to occur?'
> 'What are the benefits and how likely are they?'
> 'How long will it be before I will see improvement?'

You'll need to work with your medical care team to get the answers to most of these questions, but only you can answer the questions about what you want from any treatment and what's important to you.

For some people, it might be important to have 100% clear skin irrespective of treatment burden or medical risk. For others, it might be important to undergo treatments that don't take up too much time, even if the outcome is not as good.

What's important to you is likely to change over time and with the seasons, so it's a question you need to keep asking yourself. For example, it's more important for me to have clear skin on my legs in the summer than in the winter.

Working in partnership with your medical team

Unless you feel that what's important to you has been addressed in clinic, you aren't going to pay too much attention to the advice and information given. Your dermatologist or nurse is there to provide you with their expert advice and to work with you to make sure that you achieve what's important to you. The outcomes are likely to be better if everyone works together. There's a cost-benefit balance with all treatments, weighing the treatment outcome with the impact it has on your life. You need to work with your team to find the right balance for you. Clinicians can only understand your priorities if you communicate them at the right time.

If you have been diagnosed only recently, it's important to know that there are many treatment options to help you manage your symptoms. It's important that you communicate well with your doctor and medical team to find the plan that works for you.

It can be difficult to make decisions about treatments. The British Association of Dermatology has a decision-making tool on their website that can help you work out what's best for you. It also helps to hear about other people's experiences and online support forums can be a helpful way to learn from others and gain practical advice.

Some symptoms of psoriasis, like itching, are rarely discussed in clinic or treated (Meeuwis et al., 2012). It takes courage to address sensitive issues like psoriasis of the genitals and erectile dysfunction, but both are common. You may need to raise this yourself at a consultation if it's not addressed. You needn't feel embarrassed as it's a common symptom, but there are good sources of information about genital psoriasis online if you feel more comfortable accessing these first. (See the resources section in the Appendix to find reliable sources of information.)

It can help to write a list of what you want to discuss during your clinic appointment and show it to the specialist at the start. Check it before leaving so you know everything has been covered. Having something written down can be helpful if you feel embarrassed about talking about more difficult symptoms.

Most clinicians would agree that patient care is far better when decisions are joint and the patient themselves leads their healthcare management. This is called patient leadership, which means moving away from a traditional model of doctors vs. patients or 'them and us' and instead working collaboratively, with patient involvement not only at the individual level but also in service development.

It's not always easy to be assertive and speak up at clinic appointments, and even more courage is needed to be a voice for the wider psoriasis community, but there are online and in-person courses that can help coach you in these skills. If this is something of interest to you, have a look to see whether your healthcare centre offers an expert patient or self-management programme. Future Learn, in collaboration with NHS England, offers an online course in peer leadership which can help people develop their knowledge, skills and confidence in becoming partners in their own care.

Retaining information

It can be difficult to remember everything said to you during a clinic appointment. We're frequently bombarded with medical facts and terminology, and it's hard to take it all on board.

At a recent appointment, the doctor told me they wanted me to read about three different types of treatment to help inform my decision. They told me they had an order of preference for trying them and wanted me to consider that alongside the information I read. In my emotional state, it was hard to remember the names of the treatments, let alone their order of preference. Like most people in a clinic consultation, I can only remember a very small percentage of the information I am given. Evidence suggests that as much as 80% of the information given in a medical consultation is forgotten immediately (Kessels, 2003). Luckily, at this clinic appointment a junior doctor, with a pen, was also present to write down the names of the treatments in order.

It can help to take someone along with you to listen and remember information provided at appointments. If that's not possible, don't be afraid to take notes. You could even ask permission to record the consultation on your phone. That way, you can relisten to the conversation at home when you're feeling more relaxed. Others can listen too and help you think through your options. The British Medical

Association encourages this as a good way for people to remember and process important information.

Managing your treatment burden

A cystic fibrosis (CF) conference I attended a few years ago was focused on patient compliance and adherence. The question under consideration was, 'Why don't our patients do what we ask them to do?'

One research team took a novel approach, which has stayed with me ever since (van der Vegte et al., 2013). They asked a clinical team caring for people with CF to undergo the equivalent of the treatment plan for a young person with CF for four weeks. This involved the equivalent of oral medication, time-consuming inhaled antibiotics, journal keeping, structured rest and sporting activity.

In total, 18 clinicians, who had been encouraging the CF patients to follow a similar regimen, signed up for the study. Not one made it to the end of the study period, and they reported that one of the main difficulties was being made to feel different from other people. I realised that what we ask our CF patients to do, day in and day out, is hugely demanding even for a highly motivated and knowledgeable group of clinicians.

I'm not aware if this type of study has been repeated for dermatologists and psoriasis treatments, which can be similarly burdensome. During my first year at university, I was prescribed a topical treatment that I had to meticulously apply once a day, avoiding normal skin, leaving it on for increasing intervals and then washing off in a coal tar bath. The cream stained everything it came into contact with, so I wore an old dressing gown, tried not to touch anything and kept my fingers crossed that no one knocked on my door. I was living in student accommodation and it also stained the bath in our shared bathroom. I felt ashamed of the mess and smell of tar I left behind. I did this for weeks. When I finally stopped the treatment, my psoriasis was as bad as it had been and my skin was stained an alarming brown and purple hue. It wasn't an easy process to follow and it didn't even work. Little wonder so few of us can keep going with treatments like this.

Sometimes it doesn't feel realistic to apply thick, greasy ointment to extensive plaques (avoiding clear skin) twice a day, every day for weeks on end with little prospect of dramatic improvement. Especially when you lead a busy life. As a result, many people with psoriasis find it difficult to stick to treatment plans.

Behaviour change and adherence

One psychological theory suggests we change our behaviour by going through a series of stages. The first is pre-contemplation, where we have no intention or desire to change. For example, I might like smoking and want to keep smoking. The next stage is contemplation, where we're ambivalent about change. Returning to the example, I decide I want to give up smoking for my health, but I can easily slip back to pre-contemplation, or something might push me into the next stage (action) where I start to make changes to my behaviour. Hopefully, I begin to feel motivated and can see the benefits from the changes I've made, and this pushes me to the final stage (maintenance) where the new behaviour becomes established as part of my new routine. Sometimes, however, people end up relapsing and then move through the cycle again (Figure 13.1).

This cycle applies to all behaviour change, including adherence to treatment as you can see in the figure. People pass through one stage to the next and often go back and forth between the stages. It's important not to be too hard on yourself if you find yourself slipping back a few stages. If you're motivated, you can pick your treatment routine back up again.

Maintaining a good treatment routine

There may also be practical problems with maintaining a good treatment routine. For example, you may decide you want to do your

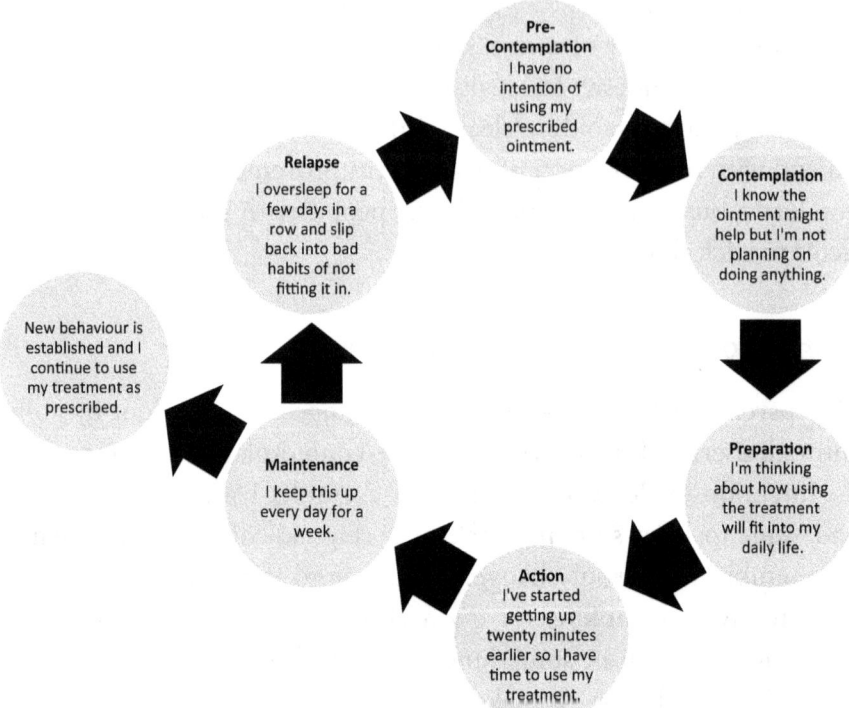

FIGURE 13.1 Cycle of behaviour change. Source: Adapted from Prochaska and DiClemente (Prochaska & DiClemente, 1983)

treatment just as your doctor has prescribed, but you're finding it difficult to remember to do it or fit it in. If that's the case, other things can help, and establishing a routine is a good place to start. It can take time for a treatment to become a habit. Some researchers have suggested it takes 21 days of consistency for a behaviour to become automatic, while others have found it can take much longer, around 70 days, depending on the behaviour.

Applying prescription moisturiser after every shower is a strong habit that I've developed over decades. It's as automatic as drying myself with a towel. This habitual behaviour goes awry when my routine is disturbed for whatever reason, but I'd say it works 95% of the time so I try not to focus on the 5% where it didn't work out.

Coping with treatments

Even if you reach a point where a behaviour is automatic, you may still benefit from reminders, especially in the early days.

> **Try this**
>
> These tricks can help you establish a good routine:
>
> 1. Set a reminder or alarm on your phone.
> 2. Use visual reminders (like Post-it notes on the fridge).
> 3. Set up systems like a box with your creams in, next to the shower.
> 4. Tie in doing treatments with your daily routine, like showering in the morning.
> 5. Sort your tablets into a Dosette box, a plastic tray in which you can sort your tablets into separate compartments for each day of the week. That way, you can see what you've taken.
> 6. Carry spare tablets in case you forget or get stuck away from home.
> 7. Decant a small amount of ointment to keep with or near you at home or work.
> 8. Pair up with a friend and start an adherence streak; make it competitive with a prize for the longest streak.
> 9. Make a motivational poster with your top five reasons for doing your treatments daily.
> 10. Use a reward system for every time you remember and treat yourself for reaching your target.

Summary

- Accepting the patient role and coming to terms with the routines and treatments that go alongside having psoriasis can be challenging.

- Treatments for psoriasis can be burdensome, and having to make decisions can be overwhelming too.
- Work with your medical team to get the best care. This means thinking about what the important outcomes for you are and communicating that to your team.
- It can be difficult to find the motivation to do treatments, but remember that behaviour changes in stages, so keep trying and don't give up.

Top tips

- Prepare for your appointments with a list of questions or topics you want to raise.
- It can be impossible to remember everything you're told during a consultation, so take notes or even record the session if that's okay with your doctor.
- If you're struggling to remember to do your treatments, try a few of the reminder strategies until you find one that works.
- Remember, if at first you don't succeed, try again. And be kind to yourself!

14 Supporting others with psoriasis

This chapter is written for people who support someone with psoriasis, including parents and other primary caregivers, partners and family members and those working in dermatological services. There are sections for each group but that's not to say the advice in each section won't be helpful for anyone in a supportive role or who lives with someone with psoriasis.

Advice for parents and other primary caregivers

Around a third of people first develop psoriasis before the age of 20. One study of children and adolescents with psoriasis (Salman et al., 2018) found that over a third of their sample rated their skin condition as having a moderate to extremely large impact on their quality of life, even when their actual symptoms were rated as mild.

Challenges for carers

Having a poor quality of life was associated with higher levels of anxiety and depression. Furthermore, the researchers discovered that the quality of life for the families of children and adolescents with psoriasis was also diminished. This means that if you care for a child or teenager with psoriasis, it is likely to affect your well-being too.

For those of you in this position, it won't be surprising news. You will be visiting clinics and hospitals with your child and helping to apply treatments, or you may be nagging older children to manage their own treatments, not to mention all the worrying that goes hand in hand with seeing your child suffer. I know there were times when my parents felt overwhelmed by not being able to 'fix it' for me.

The teenage years, a period of change and developing identity, are a particularly tough time to develop a condition that is often uncontrollable and affects appearance so greatly. Studies have shown that having psoriasis can impact an individual's life choices and interfere with their pursuit of goals, including educational attainment, family life and job or career choices (Warren et al., 2011; Kimball et al., 2005).

Whatever the age of your child with psoriasis, as a parent, it's hard to watch them struggle and you can be left feeling quite helpless.

Fortunately, there are things you can do to support your child and mitigate these effects.

Listening and providing validation

If your child comes to you upset and in distress, your instinct will be to try and fix things, cheer them up and make it right. However, at times when they're distressed, fixing is not always the first thing you should attempt to do.

There are times when looking at solutions and finding the positive in a situation can really help someone to manage their distress, but at other times it's equally important to listen, validate and help someone to process their feelings.

You can reflect back what you heard so they know you understand and that their feelings are valid: 'It sounds like things were pretty tough today and you're feeling sad'. You'll want to reassure them that it's okay to feel that way and that you're there alongside them. Empathy is different from sympathy. It's not just saying 'poor you', it's saying 'I get how hard this is and I'm here for you'. Brené Brown (Brown, 2021) describes empathy as 'understanding what people are feeling' whereas sympathy doesn't convey 'the powerful "me too" of empathy, it communicates "not me", then adds, "But I do feel sorry for you"'. Brown argues that rather than making someone feel heard and supported, sympathy can trigger feelings of shame.

Expressing the full range of emotions

You may worry that you'll make things worse by empathising and allowing them to express their emotional struggle. Remember, it's okay for your child to feel sad and frustrated by psoriasis. You don't need to shut down negative emotions as soon as they come up. Pushing negative feelings away as a long-term coping strategy has consequences for health, relationships and emotional well-being. Difficult feelings, when given free expression and properly processed, can help someone move forward and begin to develop constructive coping strategies.

The Pixar film *Inside Out* (2015) illustrates this point well with the contrast between the Joy and Sadness characters who manifest 11-year-old Riley's emotional world. Riley's life is in turmoil following a move across the country and her emotions, embodied as different characters, compete to control her feelings. There's a moment when Bing Bong, Riley's imaginary friend, sees his world collapse as Riley grows up. Joy, who has been encouraging positivity throughout the film, tries to cheer him up with tickles, silly faces and games. The Sadness character comforts Bing Bong by letting him feel his sadness at losing Riley. This comforts Bing Bong and makes him feel able to keep going. Finally, at the end of the film, Joy realises the importance of allowing Riley to feel sad; by expressing her sadness and letting others know how she feels, Riley finally gets the support and comfort she needs. This is a useful film to explain the importance of feeling all types of emotion, even the unpleasant ones. You could watch this with your child and talk about the importance of their feelings and emotions, even if it makes them feel sad for a while. It can help them to know that they don't have to pretend to be fine and put on a brave face all the time; sometimes it's okay to feel fed up.

Dealing with unwanted attention

Living with a visible skin condition will mean that people will ask your child questions, point, stare, grimace and so on. Unless you plan to keep your child at home or covered up for the rest of their lives, you can help them prepare for how to deal with unwanted attention. Teach them the Explain-Reassure-Distract method of managing comments and questions described in Chapter 5 and get them to practise until it becomes automatic.

It's also likely that people will direct their comments and questions to you. If that happens, and someone asks you what's wrong with your child's skin, you can model the same Explain-Reassure-Distract approach. This will be an opportunity for your child to learn by watching you respond in a calm way that keeps you in control of the conversation.

Managing their own care and treatments

At some point, your child will need to take responsibility for their own treatment and care. While it's natural for parents to be very involved in clinic appointments and decisions with young children, as your child approaches their teen years you can start supporting them to take greater responsibility. Your child will feel more in control of their treatment and medical care if you encourage them to speak in clinic appointments and begin to be involved in decision-making (Rasmussen et al., 2018).

We're all quite bad at following medical advice, and it will be the same for your child. Treatments take up valuable time and remind them that they're not the same as their friends. You could easily get into a battle of wills if you start to cajole them into doing treatments. Instead, try to support them to develop a treatment regimen that works for them, and remember to give lots of praise if they manage their treatments by themselves. For younger children, consider using a reward chart to help motivate them.

Supporting self-esteem

As described in earlier chapters, growing up with psoriasis may affect your child's feelings of self-esteem. There are things you can do to help build their confidence. If you notice something they're doing well, make sure you tell them. Share with them the reasons why you think they're wonderful. Are they funny, kind, clever or creative? Your child is much more than their skin condition, so remind them of that.

Don't make them show their skin to others if they don't feel ready. It might not look unsightly to you, but it takes a lot of courage to show skin covered in psoriasis to the world. If they're not ready, it may feel distressing for them. Ask yourself whether it matters if they want to wear trousers instead of shorts? You can even join them in their choice of clothing, to normalise it where appropriate.

You could help to motivate your child by watching movies with inspiring characters. Read books together where the main character has imperfections or even psoriasis. One option might be the book *Wonder* by R. J. Palacio, where the main character, Auggie, is a ten-year-old boy born with a genetic condition that affects his appearance.

Spotting warning signs

It's not always easy to tell if your child is having psychological difficulties or being bullied about their appearance, but sudden changes in behaviour might be a sign. Other indicators can include interacting less with family and friends, and changes in appetite or sleep patterns. You might notice that your child has lost interest in the things they used to enjoy or they are suddenly finding excuses not to go to school. Don't hesitate to ask for professional help if you're worried.

There's nothing more painful than seeing your child suffer and having no control. Be there for them, listen to them and support them to develop coping strategies. This will stand them in good stead throughout their lives.

If you're struggling too, then seek support for yourself; reach out to friends or join an online forum where you can meet others in the same situation. It's important to know you are not alone. Remember, too, that you could ask your GP for a referral to a counselling service, or your child's dermatology clinic might be able to refer you to a mental health professional.

Partners and other family members

If you have a partner or family member who has psoriasis and you want to support them, the first thing you should do is learn about the condition. This book will help you understand the main psychological challenges they may be facing, and there are good sources of information online such as the Psoriasis Association. See the resource section at the end of this book for good sources of information about psoriasis.

When you care about a person's well-being and you see them struggling, it's instinctive to want to make them feel better. You want to tell them that it's not so bad and that their looks are not impacted.

Although this is a perfectly natural and loving response, there is a risk that when you try to make someone feel better by challenging their thoughts, they end up feeling unheard or misunderstood, thereby invalidating their experience. At such times, it is more helpful to simply listen and recognise their feelings. Try to resist the urge to 'fix' or minimise their condition and instead acknowledge the burden and their struggles in a supportive way.

You may be able to support them in practical ways too. Someone with psoriatic arthritis (PsA) may feel ashamed about not being able to do the essential daily activities they used to and might resist asking for help. Don't be afraid to ask someone what you can do to help. Offer practical help, especially when you notice that they're struggling with a task.

Attending appointments and helping with treatment decisions could make a huge difference to your partner or family member. It helps me when someone also listens to information and advice at consultations, and I like to discuss my options with my husband before deciding on a new course of treatment.

People working in dermatology

The relationships I've had with the professionals who have looked after me over the years have been important to me. Throughout my twenties and thirties, I had regular phototherapy at the same unit in a London hospital. In my twenties, the outpatient treatment involved the application of ointment to every part of my body on a ward, followed by a coal tar bath and then UVB therapy. This was repeated three times a week and so I spent a lot of time in the company of the same nurses. They cared for me with incredible kindness and compassion, supporting me through periods of change in my life (including house moves and childbirth).

Long-term care for mind and body

It is not unusual for people with psoriasis to be seen by the same dermatology multidisciplinary team for many years, especially when having treatment like phototherapy, which requires care several times a week for months at a time.

This gives those who work in dermatology the opportunity to get to know someone at a deeper level than is normally possible in a ten-minute consultation. Therefore, it's important to think about each interaction and the opportunity you have to support people to access the best medical care.

Though you have been trained to care for a physical condition, you also have to think about an individual's psychological well-being. It's impossible to separate the mind from the body as the two are inextricably linked.

Across many physical health conditions, people in psychological distress have worse health outcomes. They miss more appointments and present at emergency services more frequently. They're more likely to have inpatient stays and, when admitted, they're more likely to stay in the hospital for a longer period, resulting in increasing healthcare costs. It's estimated that mental health difficulties alongside chronic illness cost the NHS in England between £8 billion and £13 billion a year (Naylor et al., 2012).

This means your team will not be able to treat an individual's psoriasis effectively if a patient has poorly controlled mental health difficulties. Fortunately, psychological distress can improve with the right support.

Recognising psychological distress

As discussed in Chapter 5, people with psoriasis may be avoidant of their feelings and there is an increased risk of emotional blindness or alexithymia. As a consequence, when you ask someone with psoriasis how they are, they might tell you all is well and they're fine. Even if you ask directly about how psoriasis affects their daily life, chances are they're likely to tell you it has no impact.

This is because they will have adjusted their expectations and no longer consider certain activities that others take for granted, like going for a swim, an option anymore, so it's not something they think they are missing out on.

To fully understand the impact of psoriasis on well-being, you'll need to ask patients a range of direct questions about specific aspects of daily life. You can use structured quality of life questionnaires, like the Dermatology Life Quality Index (DLQI) (Finlay & Khan, 1994), but it's important to take an interest in the responses your patient provides and ask follow-up questions about why they gave a particular answer so you can explore the meaning behind it together.

Exploring illness perceptions

Using the illness perceptions model as a framework can be another helpful way to start a discussion about the impact psoriasis has on a person's life (see Chapter 10). This model will help you understand how someone's beliefs about psoriasis are driving their emotional response to the condition, and how they are behaving and coping.

Because these beliefs are held implicitly, it's unlikely your patient will volunteer the information unless you ask direct questions such as:

- 'What do you think caused your psoriasis in the first place?'
- 'What are your symptoms?' (Here you may need to prompt with questions about skin, pain, itch, sleep, digestion, anxiety, low mood.)
- 'Does anything make your skin worse?'
- 'What helps calm things down?'
- 'How do you think your skin will be in one year from now, ten years from now, twenty years from now?'
- 'How does psoriasis affect your life?'
- 'Does it influence any choices you make?'
- 'Are there things you no longer do that you'd love to?'
- 'How much control do you have over your symptoms?'
- 'How effective are your treatments?'
- 'What are your concerns about negative effects of your treatment such as side-effects, inconvenience, cost?'

In Chapter 10, you can read the examples of how illness perceptions can drive the way a person copes with psoriasis and the impact on their feelings and behaviour.

The way you pose these questions is also important if you want to understand the impact of psoriasis on someone's life. Using closed questions (which can be answered with a yes or no) often generates a reply that's short and to the point. Open-ended questions, on the other hand, invite a longer answer and yield more information.

Closed questions can be helpful in confirming details of symptoms, but open-ended questioning is more likely to result in a greater depth of information about perceptions, emotions, motivations and barriers. Examples of open-ended alternatives to closed questions are given in Table 14.1.

TABLE 14.1 Open-ended alternatives to closed questions

Closed question	Open-ended question
Did the treatment work for you?	Tell me how you got on with the treatment?
How long have you had psoriasis?	Can you tell me about how you first got psoriasis?
Does your psoriasis itch?	Many people say their psoriasis feels itchy at times, how is that for you?
Are you feeling stressed or anxious?	Can you tell me about your stress levels at the moment?
Does psoriasis stop you from doing anything?	How does psoriasis affect your day-to-day life? Tell me about the things you might do if you didn't have psoriasis.
Are you feeling depressed?	How have you been feeling emotionally?

Reflective listening and summarising

Reflective listening is another technique for getting someone to talk in more depth. This can involve something as simple as repeating what someone has just said, but you could also paraphrase it or even use a metaphor.

A summary is a longer reflection, bringing together all the information you've just been told. It can help to focus on what the person is feeling, as opposed to their situation. For example:

> Patient: 'Nothing helps. I feel like giving up with all this treatment'.
> Healthcare professional: 'So it feels like nothing is working right now and you just want to stop your treatments. It feels like there's no light at the end of the tunnel'.

Reflections help to demonstrate that you are really listening and can encourage a patient to open up, but they also provide an opportunity to check whether you've understood something correctly.

Reflecting back on a negative emotion or situation might feel daunting. It's normal to worry that you might magnify a problem and make things worse, but that's not the case. When you know someone has really heard your distress and demonstrates that by offering a reflection or a summary, it feels comforting and is unlikely to aggravate the situation.

In my clinical practice, I've had people correct my reflections and tell me that I haven't quite understood, and then they go on to clarify and explain further. This is actually a helpful way to ensure you and your patient are talking about the same things. Reflections are an essential tool if you really want to understand the people in your care.

Approaching sensitive topics

Some topics may feel awkward to approach, like sex-related impairment and psoriasis of the genitals. People with psoriasis are unlikely to raise sensitive topics first, even though they may be experiencing significant discomfort or distress. Over a third of the people with psoriasis you see will have plaques in the anogenital area, causing problems with relationships and body image as well as itching (da Silva et al., 2020). Raising it as a topic in a clinic setting normalises the occurrence of genital psoriasis and reduces the amount of shame felt. Given the opportunity, most people with anogenital psoriasis will be relieved if invited to talk about it and get appropriate treatment.

Broadening the focus of care

Behaviour change and pursuing a healthy lifestyle are greatly emphasised in psoriasis care. The only psoriasis poster on the hospital wall where I get my phototherapy treatment is related to improving lifestyle as a way to manage symptoms (eating better, drinking less, exercising more). While this might be helpful for some people, it's important to put lifestyle choices in context and recognise the complexity of the social and environmental factors involved in health.

Determinants of health other than lifestyle factors include the physical environment, factors like air and water quality, social and economic circumstances and clinical care. The Kaiser Family Foundation estimates that only 30% of the variance in health outcomes is attributable to health behaviours, while as much as 20% is accounted for by access to, and the quality of, medical care alone (Remington et al., 2015).

As a healthcare professional, be aware of your implicit biases. It's easy to focus on things you see as part of the problem and that need fixing, like a person's weight, but it's important to be aware of other issues that may be contributing, such as healthcare inequalities based on gender, ethnicity or mental health difficulties.

Focusing only on lifestyle factors is likely to make an individual feel blamed for their psoriasis, 'They're too fat, too lazy, not good at doing their treatments'. There's a fine balance between encouraging behaviour change and victim blaming in a population that already feels shame and low self-worth.

Dealing with emotional difficulties and depression

You might prefer to stick to talking about physical problems and worry that by encouraging a patient to think about their emotional difficulties and talk about their struggles, you'll break a dam that you don't have the time, knowledge or resources to deal with. Among health professionals, it is common to feel concerned about what to do if someone cries during treatment or a clinic appointment. These are the most important things to remember:

- Emotions are not dangerous and it can be extremely helpful to express them.
- You didn't cause the distress but provided a space so it could be expressed.
- You don't need to fix it.
- You won't make things worse by responding with empathy like, 'That sounds really hard'.

- Reflections can be helpful, like, 'I can see this is really upsetting for you'.
- Don't try to shut it down by pointing out positives or encouraging bravery.
- Don't say 'I know how you feel' unless you really do. Be authentic and sincere in your responses.
- If you feel helpless, ask, 'Is there anything I can do?' Then respond with, 'Here's what I'm able to do'.

Familiarise yourself with the NICE guidelines for identifying and recognising depression in people with physical health problems (NICE, 2010). If you are concerned that someone is clinically depressed, then ask the following questions:

'During the last month, have you often been bothered by feeling down, depressed or hopeless?'
'During the last month, have you often been bothered by having little interest or pleasure in doing things?'

If the answer to either question is yes, then consider a referral to the person's general practitioner or mental health services.

There may be times when an individual expresses suicidal thoughts. If you are concerned that someone may be at immediate risk to themselves or others, refer them immediately to specialist mental health services. Seek training on how to identify risk and your place of work's protocol about how to manage it.

Finally, be aware that emotional and psychological problems won't necessarily improve as plaques and pain improve. It's often the case that people only feel they have the space to express emotional distress once their psoriasis is in remission. Even after long periods of clear skin and pain-free joints, the psychological distress, low self-esteem and shame may persist. You need to ask about psychological difficulties even in people with mild psoriasis and those in remission.

Summary

- Living with psoriasis is difficult and people you care for will often struggle.
- Feelings are not dangerous; it helps if someone is able to express their distress.
- Remember, you don't have to try to 'fix' the condition or downplay the negative experiences of people you care for. Listen, acknowledge and support instead.
- Don't be afraid to ask, 'What can I do?'
- Learn about psoriasis and get support for yourself if you need it.

Top tips

- Remember, emotions are not dangerous.
- It's important for someone in distress to be heard.
- Use reflections to show you're listening and you empathise.
- Using open questions will help you get a good understanding of someone's situation.
- Your support can help someone with psoriasis feel and cope better.

15 Positive growth and psoriasis

Growing up with psoriasis has shaped me and impacted all aspects of my life. For better or worse, it has made me who I am, how I view myself, how I relate to other people and how I cope with life's difficulties. I credit some of my skill as a psychologist working in a medical setting to the fact that I live with a chronic illness and I've had a lifetime of medical appointments and treatments.

As we have seen in previous chapters, psoriasis can have a negative impact on many areas of life. I want to end this book by thinking about the ways I've grown as a person because of my psoriasis and the manner in which I've learnt to manage the condition and its consequences.

That is not to say I'm glad I have it, or I wouldn't choose to be rid of it in an instant. I would! But I have to acknowledge that I am who I am because of, and not despite, psoriasis.

Recognising the positives

On the positive side, I've developed key strengths as a result of psoriasis, including:

- having empathy and compassion for people who live with chronic health problems, which influenced my career and benefited my professional skills;
- growing awareness of the wider benefits of a healthy lifestyle, including regular exercise, good sleep, meditation and avoiding processed foods;
- learning to navigate medical settings as a patient, asking appropriate questions, being assertive and researching treatment options;

- being aware of stress levels and learning to manage stressors effectively;
- learning to put things into perspective and not 'sweating the small stuff';
- appreciating the small pleasures in life;
- knowing my family and friends love me, whatever I look like;
- noticing my self-critical voice and being kind to myself.

Personal growth mindset

There are still times when I feel overwhelmed by psoriasis, but over the years I've learnt to cope through many small adjustments to my thinking and behaviour. If I think back to how I used to be and how I am now, I can see real differences in how I manage things, even though there are times when I don't feel like I'm coping.

Take the following example of a family wedding that I thought I handled well at the time, with my usual strategy of ignoring and hiding. It was a black-tie event and we were all looking forward to celebrating together. It's normal on such occasions for people to put a lot of thought and effort into what they wear, spending hours searching for the perfect outfit. We do this for a number of reasons: how we look communicates a great deal to the people around us; it tells the world that we honour and respect a special occasion; and looking good can help us to feel good.

At that time, I had extensive psoriasis on my arms, legs, shoulders and back, so I needed an evening dress that would send all the right social messages while covering as much of my skin as possible and not revealing flakes of skin on my back and shoulders. Unfortunately, long-sleeved, light-coloured, floor-length evening dresses were not readily available. I scoured the shops trying to find a dress that ticked all the boxes, yet still made me look good and feel fashionable. It was a frustrating search. While family members chatted excitedly about their formalwear options, the only suitable clothes I could find made me look like a nun in a habit. Despite the stress, I didn't share my difficulties with anyone and instead minimised the struggle I felt.

Eventually, I found a lovely long-sleeved wrap dress, except it was only available in black, a nightmare for showing flakes of skin on my shoulders and back, and it was knee length. After further searching, I found that tights made for ice skaters looked flesh-coloured but were in fact thick enough to withstand falls on the ice, which meant they were also thick enough to hide my skin. If you looked at me from a distance, you couldn't tell they were thick tights and I looked like I had flawless skin.

I bought the dress and resolved to cope with the flakes on my shoulders, priming my husband to keep a close eye on my appearance and surreptitiously brush away any skin he saw. Admittedly, it wasn't the perfect outfit. When I tried it on and looked at my reflection, I was convinced I looked frumpy and unfashionable. But I felt I had no other choice.

On the day of the wedding, my immediate family got ready at my parents' home. One by one, they came out in their evening dresses, full length to the floor, bare shoulders and arms. We all cooed with admiration as they swirled around in excitement, looking glamorous. And then it was my turn, in the one dress I could find that ticked some of my boxes, with itchy thick nylon tights which I prayed no-one paid too much close attention to.

I felt self-conscious and out of place, dressed more for a business lunch than a fairy-tale ball. I took myself away and sobbed, overwhelmed by pain and frustration. I had no control over my skin. I didn't look like everyone else. The shame I felt about the psoriasis on my arms and legs led me to go to such great and distressing lengths to hide it.

In the end I dried my tears, switched off my emotions, put on a smile and got on with it. What else could I do?

When I think back to this time in my life, it feels as if I was caught up in a tornado, tossed and buffeted and unable to anchor myself. I felt alone and out of control. I was unkind to myself and self-critical. Many years later, I recognise I could have done things differently.

Now, I would tell someone how I was feeling. This doesn't come easily to me after many years of keeping my feelings to myself, but I would remind myself about the importance of feeling understood and supported. If my family and friends had known how much I was struggling, they would have given me emotional support and they might have offered practical help in my search for an outfit.

I would have noticed that my beliefs at the time included 'no treatments will work', 'the situation is hopeless', 'my psoriasis is out of my control'. Instead, I would have made an appointment to see my doctor. I would have asked what my treatment options were in the months leading up to the wedding. I would have challenged any thought that I had no time for outpatient phototherapy, and I would have asked my family and friends for help getting to my appointments.

When I looked at myself on the day of the wedding, my perception was clouded by negative thoughts about my appearance and comparisons with others. With hindsight, I can see that my dress was beautiful and the only person judging me critically was myself. Instead, I would distance myself from my thoughts which were telling me that I look awful and that people will be critical of my dress. I would remind myself that these thoughts are just difficult passengers on my bus. Rather than putting my energy and all my attention into arguing or debating with these passengers, I would instead focus on the day and on spending time with the people I love. I would try to treat myself with kindness and compassion, not by ignoring my disappointment but by recognising the positive aspects of my appearance and the social occasion.

I would now recognise how stressful this episode was and make sure I took positive steps to help me feel calm and soothed. I would have meditated and made time for things I love and find fulfilling.

Above all, I would have reminded myself how well I cope with psoriasis (on the whole) and that I'm not to blame. I would have told myself it is a complex immune-mediated condition and I have nothing to feel ashamed of.

As a result, I might have decided to wear a sleeveless dress and felt confident enough to deal with any unwanted attention. I would still have had psoriasis. But instead of feeling isolated, unattractive and miserable, I would have felt supported and better about myself.

Commitments for positive living

Everyone with psoriasis should be able to live well and thrive. If you have found any of the ideas in this book useful, why not make your own resolutions for change? Writing them down can help you commit to making them a reality.

As an illustration, my own commitments for living with psoriasis are as follows:

> - I will share with my family and friends when I'm struggling.
> - I will notice when my thinking is negative and remind myself that just because I think something doesn't make it real.
> - I will focus on the things that are important to me and give my life meaning and value.
> - I will keep working with my medical team to find the treatment regimen that works best for me.
> - I will notice when I'm being self-critical and instead talk to myself with compassion.
> - I will engage in activities that help me feel soothed, content and calm.
> - I will connect with other people with psoriasis.
> - I will remind myself I'm doing my best at living with a difficult condition.

Try this

Use the space here to make your own commitments:

Appendices

Resources

Information about psoriasis

1. Psoriasis Association
   https://www.psoriasis-association.org.uk/
   The Psoriasis Association is the leading UK charity and membership organisation for people affected by psoriasis. They are a reliable source of information and advice. Members receive a quarterly magazine *Pso* with interesting articles and latest information. The Psoriasis Association raise awareness of psoriasis, fund and promote research and represent the interests of members.

2. National Psoriasis Foundation (NPF)
   https://www.psoriasis.org/
   The NPF is the leading US-based non-profit organisation supporting research on psoriasis and psoriatic arthritis and advocating for the needs of the psoriatic disease community. The mission of the NPF is to drive efforts to cure psoriatic disease and improve the lives of those affected.

3. The Psoriasis and Psoriatic Arthritis Alliance (PAPAA)
   https://www.papaa.org/
   The PAPAA is a UK-based charity founded in 2007 by merging the Psoriatic Arthropathy Alliance (PAA) and the Psoriasis Support Trust (PST). It provides multimedia information and advice including videos, written articles and digital newsletters for people with psoriasis and psoriatic arthritis.

4. Canadian Association of Psoriasis Patients (CAPP)
   https://canadianpsoriasis.ca/en/
   The CAPP mission is to raise awareness, provide education, advocate for better access to care and treatments, and support research. They produce a bilingual newsletter.

5. Psoriasis Australia
   https://psoriasisaustralia.org.au/
   Psoriasis Australia is an Australian-based charity offering information, support, advocacy and education to individuals impacted by psoriatic disease, and to their families, carers and healthcare professionals.

6. Global Psoriasis Atlas
   https://www.globalpsoriasisatlas.org/en/
   Global Psoriasis Atlas is a long-term collaborative project between three dermatology organisations: the International Federation of Psoriasis Associations, the International League of Dermatological Societies and the International Psoriasis Council. One of its main aims is to provide detailed, open-access information about the worldwide epidemiology of psoriasis.

Understanding psoriasis treatments

1. British Association of Dermatology (BAD)
   https://www.bad.org.uk/
   The BAD offers patient information leaflets about psoriasis and latest treatments. They also provide a helpful decision aid for biological therapy. https://cdn.bad.org.uk/uploads/2021/12/29200150/Decision-aid.pdf

Psoriasis support groups

1. Psoriasis Association support forums
   https://www.psoriasis-association.org.uk/forums/

2. Talk Psoriasis
   https://www.psoriasis.org/talk-psoriasis/
   National Psoriasis Association and Twill Care have partnered to provide an online community with peer support.

3. Reddit >> Psoriasis
   https://www.reddit.com/r/Psoriasis/
   A help forum about all matters relating to psoriasis including support, giving advice or looking for help.

4. The PAPAA forum
   https://www.papaa.org/get-involved/the-papaa-forum/
   The PAPAA forum is a dedicated forum discussion area for anyone with an interest in psoriasis and psoriatic arthritis to share the latest research, personal views and opinions, and talk about the natural treatments for psoriasis.

Informative videos

1. "Listening to Shame with Brené Brown"
   https://www.ted.com/talks/brene_brown_listening_to_shame?utm_campaign=tedspread&utm_medium=referral&utm_source=tedcomshare
   A powerful TED talk by shame researcher Brené Brown.

2. "Living & Dying Well Using ACT: My Life as a Clinical Psychologist with Terminal Cancer"
   https://www.sfh-tr.nhs.uk/our-services/clinical-psychology-cancer-service/dying-well-using-act-life-as-a-psychologist-with-cancer/

3. "The Secret to a Happy Life with Robert Waldinger"
   https://www.ted.com/talks/robert_waldinger_what_makes_a_good_life_lessons_from_the_longest_study_on_happiness?utm_campaign=tedspread&utm_medium=referral&utm_source=tedcomshare

A TED talk by psychiatrist Robert Waldinger about the importance of warm connections with others.

Sleep resources

1. *The Sleep Book: How to Sleep Well Every Night* by Guy Meadows

2. Sleep School
   https://www.sleepschool.org
   Sleep School is recommended by the NHS, amongst others. It aims to help individuals overcome their sleeping problems and sleeping better, for life. There's a free seven-day trial and then a subscription fee.

3. Insomnia Coach
   https://insomniacoach.com/
   Insomnia Coach is a free app created for everyone to help manage insomnia. The app is based on Cognitive Behavioral Therapy for Insomnia (CBT-I).

Appearance concerns support

1. Changing Faces
   https://www.changingfaces.org.uk
   Changing Faces is a Visible Difference and Disfigurement Charity aiming to help everyone in the UK who has a visible difference, a scar, mark or condition on their face or body that makes them look different. They have lots of helpful information and resources.

2. Appearance Matters
   https://www.uwe.ac.uk/research/centres-and-groups/appearance/resources
   Appearance Matters podcast from the Centre for Appearance Research; the world's largest research group focusing on the role of appearance and body image in people's lives.

Psychological interventions

More information about the therapeutic techniques described in this book.

1. Mindfulness
   The Velindre Mindfulness App
   https://play.google.com/store/apps/details?id=com.velindrecc.mindfulness&hl=en_GB
   The Velindre Mindfulness App was developed by the psychology team at the Velindre Cancer Centre but is deliberately non-cancer specific so that anyone can use the app to manage stress and anxiety.

   Palouse Mindfulness
   https://palousemindfulness.com
   Palouse Mindfulness is a freely available online eight-week mindfulness-based stress reduction course with worksheets, audio-guided meditations and videos.

   Headspace
   https://www.headspace.com/mindfulness
   Headspace is a widely used mindfulness app that can help you practise mindfulness. There is a free trial when you download the app.

2. ACT
   ACT Mindfully
   https://www.actmindfully.com.au/
   ACT Mindfully offers more information, resources and workshops.

   The Happiness Trap by Russ Harris

3. CFT
   The Compassionate Mind Foundation
   https://www.compassionatemind.co.uk/
   The Compassionate Mind Foundation offers lots of information and free resources about developing self-compassion.

Self-Compassion by Kristin Neff
https://self-compassion.org/
The Self-Compassion website has lots of free resources for developing self-compassion.

4. CBT
British Association for Behavioural and Cognitive Psychotherapies
https://babcp.com/
Information about CBT and a register of CBT practitioners.

5. IPT
Interpersonal Psychotherapy UK Network
https://www.iptuk.net/
Information about IPT and register of IPT practitioners in the UK.

Defeating Depression: How to Use the People in Your Life to Open the Door to Recovery by Roslyn Law

6. *Maybe You Should Talk to Someone* by Lori Gottlieb explores the process of psychotherapy through her experience as a therapist and patient.

Mental health concerns

For some people, a diagnosis of psoriasis can lead to or exacerbate mental health difficulties, such as anxiety disorders or depression. Whilst you may experience many of the symptoms below after your diagnosis and during your treatment, there may be cause for concern **if these persist**.

Symptoms of Depression:

- feeling down or hopeless;
- little interest or pleasure in things you usually enjoy;
- feeling bad about yourself;
- feeling irritable;
- feeling tired, lacking energy;
- difficulty concentrating;
- difficulty sleeping, or wanting to sleep all the time;
- loss of appetite or overeating;
- thoughts of suicide or of not wanting to be around.

Symptoms of Anxiety

- feeling nervous or anxious;
- difficulty relaxing;
- ongoing worrying thoughts;
- worrying about many different things;

- fearing the worst;
- feeling irritable;
- feeling restless or agitated.

If you find you are experiencing several of these symptoms persistently, you should seek further help. Please do not feel you need to try to cope on your own. There is help available. It is also important that you let a family member or friend know how you are feeling so that they can help you to access the support you need and hopefully be available as an additional source of support.

Where to seek further support

1. Your dermatology team may have access to a clinical, counselling or health psychologist. These are highly trained and regulated practitioner psychologists who are trained to work with people struggling with the emotional impact of physical health problems. If you are experiencing significant emotional difficulties, then you may be referred to a psychologist.
2. Your GP will have the best knowledge of what general mental health support is available in your area. Some people find it difficult to approach their GP as they perhaps don't see one GP regularly, or find it difficult to actually get an appointment. But it is really important that you reach out in relation to mental health difficulties.
3. In England, you should be able to self-refer to your local Improving Access to Psychological Therapies (IAPT) service. These services offer short-term counselling and therapies to people experiencing common mental health difficulties. More information can be found on the NHS website.
4. If you wish to see a psychologist privately, it is important to ensure you see someone who is highly trained and regulated. The term 'psychologist' is not a protected title. Therefore, you should seek someone who is registered with the Health and

Care Professions Council (HCPC). Anyone calling themselves a clinical, health or counselling psychologist should be registered with HCPC. You can check the register on the HCPC website. For more on finding a clinical psychologist, the Association of Clinical Psychologists UK (ACP-UK) has a useful guide on its website.

If you are at risk to yourself

For some people living with psoriasis, thoughts of self-harm or that you would be better off dead can become more frequent and concerning. As stated above, thoughts of suicide or not wanting to be around can be an indication of depression. If you notice **any of the below** symptoms, then you should seek immediate help:

- being preoccupied with thoughts of death or dying;
- making a plan of how you would end your life;
- taking steps to say goodbye to loved ones;
- acquiring things to follow through your plan;
- writing a suicide note.

Where to seek further crisis support

1. It is important to let your GP know about any of these symptoms. Ask for an urgent appointment.
2. If you live in the UK, you can call NHS 111 and select Option 2 if you need urgent mental health care, but it's not life threatening. This telephone line is available 24 hours a day, 7 days a week. It is free to call from a landline and mobile and if the caller has no credit.
3. The Samaritans are trained to support people who are feeling suicidal. You can call them for free at any time on 116 123. There are also other ways to get in touch with the Samaritans on their website.

4. If you are concerned that you are at high or immediate risk of suicide, then you should go to the Accident & Emergency Department at your local hospital. There will be a psychiatric liaison team on duty who will be able to assess you and work with you to develop an immediate plan to support you.

Letter to my younger self

Dear Catherine (aged 16),

I know things are tough for you right now. Sore and flaky patches of psoriasis cover your body and scalp, and your nails are pitted and painful. You struggle to hide the patches on your neck and face. You feel hopeless because nothing seems to be working.

Let me help. I want to share with you some of the things I've learnt over the years about coping with psoriasis.

I'm a clinical psychologist who's worked for many years with people with all sorts of health conditions, from cleft lip to cystic fibrosis, so I know a thing or two about coping with illness.

First of all, you're not doing anything wrong. You're not eating the wrong food, you're not dealing with stress badly, you take care of yourself just right. Psoriasis is an autoimmune disease. It's not your fault.

You feel ashamed of yourself, but you're so much more than skin. You're kind and creative, and your mind is sharp and enquiring. Remind yourself what others love about you. Keep doing all the things that make you happy. Ride your horse, read, bake, giggle with your friends. You may not believe this, but soon you'll discover that exercise, especially running, is a fantastic way to cope.

You keep your sadness to yourself and that doesn't help. Tell someone how you're feeling. You worry you'll burden them, but it feels very lonely not to be understood. People love you and want to support you, so be open about your struggles. It's okay not to be okay. Living with psoriasis is hard.

It's also okay to feel upset when people point and ask you what's wrong with your skin. They'll keep doing it your whole life, so you'll need to be prepared. Have an explanation rehearsed for those moments. Something simple and to the point, and then don't be afraid to change the subject away from psoriasis. You can learn how to take control of a conversation. It's surprisingly easy and you won't feel so stressed by the unwanted attention. And that boy who touches a plaque on your leg to make his friends shriek and laugh, that was horrible, but remember most people aren't so mean. You'll learn that others are often focused more on themselves than you.

Please don't give up hope. There are treatments that can help you keep things under control. Do your best to follow your doctor's advice and instructions. It's a hassle but will make all the difference. This is really important: you need to moisturise every day; I repeat: every single day.

Catherine, I'm not going to pretend this is going to be easy but you can do it. Some days will be hard and it will feel like too much, but you'll pick yourself up and keep going. You'll become resilient and courageous, and your empathy will know no bounds. You've got so many exciting times ahead of you. Psoriasis won't stop you from having an amazing life.

Love,
Catherine (aged 50)

References

Aberer, E., Hiebler-Ragger, M., Zenker, M., Weger, W., Hofer, A., & Unterrainer, H. F. (2020). Facets of shame are differently expressed in dermatological disease: A prospective observational study. *British Journal of Dermatology*, *183*(1), 169–171. https://doi.org/10.1111/bjd.18899

Akamine, A. A., Rusch, G. D. S., Nisihara, R., & Skare, T. L. (2021). Adverse childhood experiences in patients with psoriasis. *Trends in Psychiatry and Psychotherapy*. https://doi.org/10.47626/2237-6089-2021-0251

Alexis, A. F., & Blackcloud, P. (2014). Psoriasis in skin of color: epidemiology, genetics, clinical presentation, and treatment nuances. *The Journal of Clinical and Aesthetic Dermatology*, *7*(11), 16–24.

Almeida, V., Leite, Â., Constante, D., Correia, R., Almeida, I. F., Teixeira, M., Vidal, D. G., Sousa, H. F. P. E., Dinis, M. A. P., & Teixeira, A. (2020). The mediator role of body image-related cognitive fusion in the relationship between disease severity perception, acceptance and psoriasis disability. *Behavioral Sciences (Basel, Switzerland)*, *10*(9). https://doi.org/10.3390/bs10090142

Anstey, A., McAteer, H., Kamath, N., & Percival, F. (2012). Extending psychosocial assessment of patients with psoriasis in the UK, using a self-rated, web-based survey. *Clinical and Experimental Dermatology*, *37*(7), 735–740. https://doi.org/10.1111/j.1365-2230.2012.04457.x

Armstrong, A. W., Koning, J. W., Rowse, S., Tan, H., Mamolo, C., & Kaur, M. (2017). Under-treatment of patients with moderate to severe psoriasis in the United States: Analysis of medication usage with health plan data. *Dermatology and Therapy*, *7*(1), 97–109. https://doi.org/10.1007/s13555-016-0153-2

Bartholomew, E., Chung, M., Yeroushalmi, S., Hakimi, M., Bhutani, T., & Liao, W. (2022). Mindfulness and meditation for psoriasis: A systematic review. *Dermatology and Therapy*, *12*(10), 2273–2283. https://doi.org/10.1007/s13555-022-00802-1

Berg, M., Svensson, M., Brandberg, M., & Nordlind, K. (2008). Psoriasis and stress: A prospective study. *Journal of the European Academy of Dermatology and Venereology, 22*(6), 670–674. https://doi.org/10.1111/j.1468-3083.2008.02642.x

Blome, C., Gosau, R., Radtke, M. A., Reich, K., Rustenbach, S. J., Spehr, C., Thaçi, D., & Augustin, M. (2016). Patient-relevant treatment goals in psoriasis. *Archives of Dermatological Research, 308*(2), 69–78. https://doi.org/10.1007/s00403-015-1613-8

Brown, B. (2006). Shame resilience theory: A grounded theory study on women and shame. *Families in Society: The Journal of Contemporary Social Services, 87*(1), 43–52. https://doi.org/10.1606/1044-3894.3483

Brown, B. (2021). *Atlas of the heart: Mapping meaningful connection and the language of human experience*. Vermilion.

Cacioppo, J. T., Cacioppo, S., & Gollan, J. K. (2014). The negativity bias: Conceptualization, quantification, and individual differences. *Behavioral and Brain Sciences, 37*(3), 309–310. https://doi.org/10.1017/S0140525X13002537

Cameron, K., Ogrodniczuk, J., & Hadjipavlou, G. (2014). Changes in alexithymia following psychological intervention. *Harvard Review of Psychiatry, 22*(3), 162–178. https://doi.org/10.1097/HRP.0000000000000036

Chaudhury, S., Das, A. L., John, R. T., & Ramadasan, P. (1998). Psychological factors in psoriasis. *Indian Journal of Psychiatry, 40*(3), 295–299.

Cherrez-Ojeda, I., Vanegas, E., Felix, M., Cherrez, S., Suárez-Almendariz, D., Ponton, J., Preciado, V., Ollague-Cordova, E., & Loayza, E. (2019). Alexithymia in patients with psoriasis: A cross-sectional study from ecuador. *Psychology Research and Behavior Management, 12*, 1121–1126. https://doi.org/10.2147/PRBM.S227021

da Silva, N., Augustin, M., Langenbruch, A., Mrowietz, U., Reich, K., Thaçi, D., Boehncke, W.-H., Kirsten, N., Danckworth, A., & Sommer, R. (2020). Sex-related impairment and patient needs/benefits in anogenital psoriasis: Difficult-to-communicate topics and their impact on patient-centred care. *PLOS One, 15*(7), e0235091. https://doi.org/10.1371/journal.pone.0235091

Dahlgren, G., & Whitehead, M. (2021). The Dahlgren-Whitehead model of health determinants: 30 years on and still chasing rainbows. *Public Health, 199*, 20–24. https://doi.org/10.1016/j.puhe.2021.08.009

Dana, D. (2018). *The Polyvagal Theory in Therapy Engaging the Rhythm of Regulation*. WW Norton & Co, New York and London.

Danese, A., Pariante, C. M., Caspi, A., Taylor, A., & Poulton, R. (2007). Childhood maltreatment predicts adult inflammation in a life-course study. *Proceedings of the National Academy of Sciences, 104*(4), 1319–1324. https://doi.org/10.1073/pnas.0610362104

del Molino Sergio, (translated by Bunstead Thomas). (2022). *Skin* (1st ed.). Polity Press.

Dolezal, L., & Lyons, B. (2017). Health-related shame: An affective determinant of health? *Medical Humanities, 43*(4), 257–263. https://doi.org/10.1136/medhum-2017-011186

References

Elise Kleyn, C., McKie, S., Ross, A. R., Montaldi, D., Gregory, L. J., Elliott, R., Isaacs, C. L., Anderson, I. M., Richards, H. L., William Deakin, J. F., Fortune, D. G., & Griffiths, C. E. M. (2009). Diminished neural and cognitive responses to facial expressions of disgust in patients with psoriasis: A functional magnetic resonance imaging study. *Journal of Investigative Dermatology, 129*(11), 2613–2619. https://doi.org/10.1038/jid.2009.152

Ely, P. H. (2018). Is psoriasis a bowel disease? Successful treatment with bile acids and bioflavonoids suggests it is. *Clinics in Dermatology, 36*(3), 376–389. https://doi.org/10.1016/j.clindermatol.2018.03.011

Esposito, M., Saraceno, R., Giunta, A., Maccarone, M., & Chimenti, S. (2006). An Italian study on psoriasis and depression. *Dermatology, 212*(2), 123–127. https://doi.org/10.1159/000090652

Fabrazzo, M., Romano, F., Arrigo, M., Puca, R. V., Fuschillo, A., de Santis, V., Sampogna, G., Giordano, G. M., Catapano, F., & lo Schiavo, A. (2022). A multivariate analysis of depression prevalence in psoriasis patients: A cohort study. *International Journal of Environmental Research and Public Health, 19*(4), 2060. https://doi.org/10.3390/ijerph19042060

Finlay, A. Y., & Khan, G. K. (1994). Dermatology Life Quality Index (DLQI)-a simple practical measure for routine clinical use. *Clinical and Experimental Dermatology, 19*(3), 210–216. https://doi.org/10.1111/j.1365-2230.1994.tb01167.x

Ford, A. R., Siegel, M., Bagel, J., Cordoro, K. M., Garg, A., Gottlieb, A., Green, L. J., Gudjonsson, J. E., Koo, J., Lebwohl, M., Liao, W., Mandelin, A. M., Markenson, J. A., Mehta, N., Merola, J. F., Prussick, R., Ryan, C., Schwartzman, S., Siegel, E. L., … Armstrong, A. W. (2018). Dietary recommendations for adults with psoriasis or psoriatic arthritis from the medical board of the National Psoriasis Foundation. *JAMA Dermatology, 154*(8), 934. https://doi.org/10.1001/jamadermatol.2018.1412

Gilbert, P. (2010). *The compassionate mind: A new approach to Life's challenges.* New Harbinger Pubns Inc.

Gilbert, P. (2014). The origins and nature of compassion focused therapy. *British Journal of Clinical Psychology, 53*(1), 6–41. https://doi.org/10.1111/bjc.12043

Gottlieb, L. (2019). *Maybe you should talk to someone.* Scribe Publications.

Green, A., Shaddick, G., Charlton, R., Snowball, J., Nightingale, A., Smith, C., Tillett, W., & McHugh, N. (2020). Modifiable risk factors and the development of psoriatic arthritis in people with psoriasis. *British Journal of Dermatology, 182*(3), 714–720. https://doi.org/10.1111/bjd.18227

Griffiths, C. E. M., Augustin, M., Naldi, L., Romiti, R., Guevara-Sangines, E., Howe, T., Pietri, G., Gilloteau, I., Richardson, C., Tian, H., & Jo, S. J. (2018). Patient-dermatologist agreement in psoriasis severity, symptoms and satisfaction: Results from a real-world multinational survey. *Journal of the European Academy of Dermatology and Venereology, 32*(9), 1523–1529. https://doi.org/10.1111/jdv.14937

References

Gupta, M. A., & Gupta, A. K. (1995). The Psoriasis Life Stress Inventory: A preliminary index of psoriasis-related stress. *Acta Dermato-Venereologica*, *75*(3), 240–243. https://doi.org/10.2340/0001555575240243

Hawro, M., Maurer, M., Weller, K., Maleszka, R., Zalewska-Janowska, A., Kaszuba, A., Gerlicz-Kowalczuk, Z., & Hawro, T. (2017). Lesions on the back of hands and female gender predispose to stigmatization in patients with psoriasis. *Journal of the American Academy of Dermatology*, *76*(4), 648-654.e2. https://doi.org/10.1016/j.jaad.2016.10.040

Hejdenberg, J., & Andrews, B. (2011). The relationship between shame and different types of anger: A theory-based investigation. *Personality and Individual Differences*, *50*(8), 1278–1282. https://doi.org/10.1016/j.paid.2011.02.024

Hewitt, R. M., Bundy, C., Newi, A., Chachos, E., Sommer, R., Kleyn, C. E., Augustin, M., Griffiths, C. E. M., & Blome, C. (2022). How do dermatologists' personal models inform a patient-centred approach to management: A qualitative study using the example of prescribing a new treatment (apremilast)*. *British Journal of Dermatology*, *187*(1), 82–88. https://doi.org/10.1111/bjd.21029

Hofmann, S. G., Grossman, P., & Hinton, D. E. (2011). Loving-kindness and compassion meditation: Potential for psychological interventions. *Clinical Psychology Review*, *31*(7), 1126–1132. https://doi.org/10.1016/j.cpr.2011.07.003

Holt-Lunstad, J., Smith, T. B., & Layton, J. B. (2010). Social relationships and mortality risk: A meta-analytic review. *PLOS Medicine*, *7*(7), e1000316. https://doi.org/10.1371/journal.pmed.1000316

Homayoon, D., Hiebler-Ragger, M., Zenker, M., Weger, W., Unterrainer, H., & Aberer, E. (2020). Relationship between skin shame, psychological distress and quality of life in patients with psoriasis: A pilot study. *Acta Dermato-Venereologica*, *100*(14), adv00205. https://doi.org/10.2340/00015555-3563

Huang, R., Wang, K., & Hu, J. (2016). Effect of probiotics on depression: A systematic review and meta-analysis of randomized controlled trials. *Nutrients*, *8*(8), 483. https://doi.org/10.3390/nu8080483

John, U. (1985). *Problems and other stories*. Fawcett cress.

Jowett, S., & Ryan, T. (1985). Skin disease and handicap: An analysis of the impact of skin conditions. *Social Science and Medicine (1982)*, *20*(4), 425–429. https://doi.org/10.1016/0277-9536(85)90021-8

Kabat-Zinn, J., Wheeler, E., Light, T., Skillings, A., Scharf, M. J., Cropley, T. G., Hosmer, D., & Bernhard, J. D. (1998). Influence of a mindfulness meditation-based stress reduction intervention on rates of skin clearing in patients with moderate to severe psoriasis undergoing photo therapy (UVB) and photochemotherapy (PUVA). *Psychosomatic Medicine*, *60*(5), 625–632. https://doi.org/10.1097/00006842-199809000-00020

References

Kamiya, K., Kishimoto, M., Sugai, J., Komine, M., & Ohtsuki, M. (2019). Risk factors for the development of psoriasis. *International Journal of Molecular Sciences*, *20*(18), 4347. https://doi.org/10.3390/ijms20184347

Kessels, R. P. C. (2003). Patients' memory for medical information. *JRSM*, *96*(5), 219–222. https://doi.org/10.1258/jrsm.96.5.219

Khullar, D. (2016, December 22). How social isolation is killing us. *New York Times*.

Kimball, A. B., Jacobson, C., Weiss, S., Vreeland, M. G., & Wu, Y. (2005). The psychosocial burden of psoriasis. *American Journal of Clinical Dermatology*, *6*(6), 383–392. https://doi.org/10.2165/00128071-200506060-00005

Kleck, R. E., & Strenta, A. C. (1985). Gender and Responses to Disfigurement in Self and Others. *Journal of Social and Clinical Psychology*, *3*(3), 257–267. https://doi.org/10.1521/jscp.1985.3.3.257

Koo, J., Marangell, L. B., Nakamura, M., Armstrong, A., Jeon, C., Bhutani, T., & Wu, J. J. (2017). Depression and suicidality in psoriasis: Review of the literature including the cytokine theory of depression. *Journal of the European Academy of Dermatology and Venereology*, *31*(12), 1999–2009. https://doi.org/10.1111/jdv.14460

Krueger, G. G., & Duvic, M. (1994). Epidemiology of Psoriasis: Clinical Issues. *Journal of Investigative Dermatology*, *102*(6), 14S-18S. https://doi.org/10.1111/1523-1747.ep12386079

Kumar, S., Flood, K., Golbari, N. M., Charrow, A. P., Porter, M. L., & Kimball, A. B. (2021). Psoriasis: Knowledge, attitudes and perceptions among primary care providers. *Journal of the American Academy of Dermatology*, *84*(5), 1421–1423. https://doi.org/10.1016/j.jaad.2020.05.151

Kuznetsova, D. (2012). *Healthy places: Councils leading on public health*. London: New Local Government Netowrk.

Lahousen, T., Kupfer, J., Gieler, U., Hofer, A., Linder, M., & Schut, C. (2014). Differences between psoriasis patients and skin-healthy controls concerning appraisal of touching, shame and disgust. *Acta Dermato–Venereologica*. https://doi.org/10.2340/00015555-2373

Łakuta, P. (2021). Brief self-affirmation intervention for adults with psoriasis for reducing anxiety and depression and boosting well-being: Evidence from a randomized controlled trial. *Psychological Medicine*, 1–11. https://doi.org/10.1017/S0033291721004499

Leo Innovation Lab. (2018). The psoriasis happiness study: People with self-reported psoriasis have a significantly reduced emotional well-being and a large happiness gap compared with fellow citizens. *Journal of the American Academy of Dermatology*, *79*(3), AB291. https://doi.org/10.1016/j.jaad.2018.05.1150

Leventhal, H., Phillips, L. A., & Burns, E. (2016). The Common-Sense Model of Self-Regulation (CSM): A dynamic framework for understanding illness self-management. *Journal of Behavioral Medicine, 39*(6), 935–946. https://doi.org/10.1007/s10865-016-9782-2

Lewis-Beck, C., Abouzaid, S., Xie, L., Baser, O., & Kim, E. (2013). Analysis of the relationship between psoriasis symptom severity and quality of life, work productivity, and activity impairment among patients with moderate-to-severe psoriasis using structural equation modeling. *Patient Preference and Adherence, 7*, 199–205. https://doi.org/10.2147/PPA.S39887

Ljosaa, T. M., Mork, C., Stubhaug, A., Moum, T., & Wahl, A. K. (2012). Skin pain and skin discomfort is associated with quality of life in patients with psoriasis. *Journal of the European Academy of Dermatology and Venereology, 26*(1), 29–35. https://doi.org/10.1111/j.1468-3083.2011.04000.x

Ljosaa, T., Rustoen, T., Mørk, C., Stubhaug, A., Miaskowski, C., Paul, S., & Wahl, A. (2010). Skin pain and discomfort in psoriasis: An exploratory study of symptom prevalence and characteristics. *Acta Dermato-Venereologica, 90*(1), 39–45. https://doi.org/10.2340/00015555-0764

Lomholt, G. (1964). Prevalence of skin diseases in a population; a census study from the Faroe Islands. *Danish Medical Bulletin, 11*, 1–7.

Luminet, O., Zech, E., Rimé, B., & Wagner, H. (2000). Predicting cognitive and social consequences of emotional episodes: The contribution of emotional intensity, the five factor model, and alexithymia. *Journal of Research in Personality, 34*(4), 471–497. https://doi.org/10.1006/jrpe.2000.2286

Magin, P., Adams, J., Heading, G., Pond, D., & Smith, W. (2008). Experiences of appearance-related teasing and bullying in skin diseases and their psychological sequelae: results of a qualitative study. *Scandinavian Journal of Caring Sciences, 22*(3), 430–436. https://doi.org/10.1111/j.1471-6712.2007.00547.x

Makeev, V. D. (1976). Complex treatment of psoriasis. *Vestnik Dermatologii i Venerologii, 4*(4), 58–61.

Martin, M. L., Gordon, K., Pinto, L., Bushnell, D. M., Chau, D., & Viswanathan, H. N. (2015). The experience of pain and redness in patients with moderate to severe plaque psoriasis. *Journal of Dermatological Treatment, 26*(5), 401–405. https://doi.org/10.3109/09546634.2014.996514

Mann D. (2013). Psoriasis and bullying: breaking the cycle. *Everyday Health.*

Mathew, A. J., & Chandran, V. (2020a). Depression in psoriatic arthritis: Dimensional aspects and link with systemic inflammation. *Rheumatology and Therapy, 7*(2), 287–300. https://doi.org/10.1007/s40744-020-00207-6

Mathew, A. J., & Chandran, V. (2020b). Depression in psoriatic arthritis: Dimensional aspects and link with systemic inflammation. *Rheumatology and Therapy, 7*(2), 287–300. https://doi.org/10.1007/s40744-020-00207-6

Meeuwis, K. A. P., van de Kerkhof, P. C. M., Massuger, L. F. A. G., de Hullu, J. A., & van Rossum, M. M. (2012). Patients' experience of psoriasis in the genital area. *Dermatology (Basel, Switzerland), 224*(3), 271–276. https://doi.org/10.1159/000338858

References

Misery, L., Shourick, J., & Taieb, C. (2020). Skin pain and psoriasis. *Journal of the American Academy of Dermatology*, *83*(1), 245–246. https://doi.org/10.1016/j.jaad.2019.12.066

Nathanson, D. (1997). Affect theory and the compass of shame. In M. Lansky & A. Morrison (Eds.), *The widening scope of shame*. Analytic Press339–354.

Naylor, C., Parsonage, M., McDaid, D., Knapp, M., Fossey, M., & Galea, A. (2012). *Long-term conditions and mental health: The cost of co-morbidities*. London: King's Fund.

NICE. (2010). *Depression in adults with a chronic physical health problem*, 1st ed. Rcpsych Publications.

O'Leary, C. J., Creamer, D., Higgins, E., & Weinman, J. (2004). Perceived stress, stress attributions and psychological distress in psoriasis. *Journal of Psychosomatic Research*, *57*(5), 465–471. https://doi.org/10.1016/j.jpsychores.2004.03.012

Ohata, C., Ohyama, B., Kuwahara, F., Katayama, E., & Nakama, T. (2019). Fingernail involvement is a bigger burden than face and scalp involvement in patients with psoriasis. *Journal of Psoriasis and Psoriatic Arthritis*, *4*(1), 28–30. https://doi.org/10.1177/2475530318806256

Padesky, C. A. (1994). Schema change processes in cognitive therapy. *Clinical Psychology and Psychotherapy*, *1*(5), 267–278. https://doi.org/10.1002/cpp.5640010502

Parisi, R., Webb, R. T., Carr, M. J., Moriarty, K. J., Kleyn, C. E., Griffiths, C. E. M., & Ashcroft, D. M. (2017). Alcohol-related mortality in patients with psoriasis. *JAMA Dermatology*, *153*(12), 1256. https://doi.org/10.1001/jamadermatol.2017.3225

Partridge, J., & Pearson, A. (2008). Don't worry…it's the inside that counts. *The Psychologist*, *21*, *21*, 490–491.

Pearl, R. L., Wan, M. T., Takeshita, J., & Gelfand, J. M. (2019). Stigmatizing attitudes toward persons with psoriasis among laypersons and medical students. *Journal of the American Academy of Dermatology*, *80*(6), 1556–1563. https://doi.org/10.1016/j.jaad.2018.08.014

Pennebaker, J., Zech, E., & Rimé, B. (2001). Disclosing and sharing emotion: Psychological, social and health consequences. In M. Stroebe, W. Stroebe, R. O. Hansson, & H. Schut (Eds.), *Handbook of bereavement research: Consequences, coping, and care* (pp. 517–539). American Psychological Association.

Picardi, A., Mazzotti, E., Gaetano, P., Cattaruzza, M. S., Baliva, G., Melchi, C. F., Biondi, M., & Pasquini, P. (2005). Stress, social support, emotional regulation, and exacerbation of diffuse plaque psoriasis. *Psychosomatics*, *46*(6), 556–564. https://doi.org/10.1176/appi.psy.46.6.556

Plutchik, R. (1980). A general psychoevolutionary theory of emotion. In *Theories of emotion* (pp. 3–33). Elsevier. https://doi.org/10.1016/B978-0-12-558701-3.50007-7

References

Porges, S. W. (2009). The polyvagal theory: New insights into adaptive reactions of the autonomic nervous system. *Cleveland Clinic Journal of Medicine, 76*(4 Suppl. 2), S86–S90. https://doi.org/10.3949/ccjm.76.s2.17

Potter, D. (1994). *Seeing the blossom*. Dennis Potter.

Prochaska, J. O., & DiClemente, C. C. (1983). Stages and processes of self-change of smoking: Toward an integrative model of change. *Journal of Consulting and Clinical Psychology, 51*(3), 390–395. https://doi.org/10.1037/0022-006X.51.3.390

Rasmussen, G. S., Kragballe, K., Maindal, H. T., & Lomborg, K. (2018). Experience of being young with psoriasis: Self-management support needs. *Qualitative Health Research, 28*(1), 73–86. https://doi.org/10.1177/1049732317737311

Remington, P. L., Catlin, B. B., & Gennuso, K. P. (2015). The county health rankings: Rationale and methods. *Population Health Metrics, 13*(1), 11. https://doi.org/10.1186/s12963-015-0044-2

Rousset, L., & Halioua, B. (2018). Stress and psoriasis. *International Journal of Dermatology, 57*(10), 1165–1172. https://doi.org/10.1111/ijd.14032

Ruble, D. N. (1977). Premenstrual symptoms: A reinterpretation. *Science, 197*(4300), 291–292. https://doi.org/10.1126/science.560058

Rucević, I., Perl, A., Barisić-Drusko, V., & Adam-Perl, M. (2003). The role of the low energy diet in psoriasis vulgaris treatment. *Collegium Antropologicum, 27*(Suppl. 1), 41–48.

Sahi, F. M., Masood, A., Danawar, N. A., Mekaiel, A., & Malik, B. H. (2020). Association between psoriasis and depression: A traditional review. *Cureus*. https://doi.org/10.7759/cureus.9708

Salman, A., Yucelten, A. D., Sarac, E., Saricam, M. H., & Perdahli-Fis, N. (2018). Impact of psoriasis in the quality of life of children, adolescents and their families: A cross-sectional study. *Anais Brasileiros de Dermatologia, 93*(6), 819–823. https://doi.org/10.1590/abd1806-4841.20186981

Sampogna, F., Puig, L., Spuls, P., Girolomoni, G., Radtke, M. A., Kirby, B., Brunori, M., Bergmans, P., Smirnov, P., Rundle, J., Castiglia, A., Lavie, F., & Paul, C. (2019). Reversibility of alexithymia with effective treatment of moderate-to-severe psoriasis: Longitudinal data from EPIDEPSO. *British Journal of Dermatology, 180*(2), 397–403. https://doi.org/10.1111/bjd.17259

Sampogna, F., Tabolli, S., & Abeni, D. (2012). Living with psoriasis: Prevalence of shame, anger, worry, and problems in daily activities and social life. *Acta Dermato-Venereologica, 92*(3), 299–303. https://doi.org/10.2340/00015555-1273

Scharloo, M., Kaptein, A. A., Weinman, J., Bergman, W., Vermeer, B. J., & Rooijmans, H. G. M. (2000). Patients' illness perceptions and coping as predictors of functional status in psoriasis: A 1-year follow-up. *British Journal of Dermatology, 142*(5), 899–907. https://doi.org/10.1046/j.1365-2133.2000.03469.x

References

Schmitt-Egenolf, M. (2016). Physical activity and lifestyle improvement in the management of psoriasis. *British Journal of Dermatology, 175*(3), 452–453. https://doi.org/10.1111/bjd.14899

Shah, R., & Bewley, A. (2014). Psoriasis: 'The badge of shame'. A case report of a psychological intervention to reduce and potentially clear chronic skin disease. *Clinical and Experimental Dermatology, 39*(5), 600–603. https://doi.org/10.1111/ced.12339

Sikora, M., Stec, A., Chrabaszcz, M., Knot, A., Waskiel-Burnat, A., Rakowska, A., Olszewska, M., & Rudnicka, L. (2020). Gut microbiome in psoriasis: An updated review. *Pathogens, 9*(6), 463. https://doi.org/10.3390/pathogens9060463

Singh, S., Taylor, C., Kornmehl, H., & Armstrong, A. W. (2017). Psoriasis and suicidality: A systematic review and meta-analysis. *Journal of the American Academy of Dermatology, 77*(3), 425-440.e2. https://doi.org/10.1016/j.jaad.2017.05.019

Snast, I., Reiter, O., Atzmony, L., Leshem, Y. A., Hodak, E., Mimouni, D., & Pavlovsky, L. (2018). Psychological stress and psoriasis: A systematic review and meta-analysis. *British Journal of Dermatology, 178*(5), e363–e363. https://doi.org/10.1111/bjd.16620

Snekvik, I., Smith, C. H., Nilsen, T. I. L., Langan, S. M., Modalsli, E. H., Romundstad, P. R., & Saunes, M. (2017). Obesity, waist circumference, weight change, and risk of incident psoriasis: Prospective data from the HUNT study. *Journal of Investigative Dermatology, 137*(12), 2484–2490. https://doi.org/10.1016/j.jid.2017.07.822

Snyder, A. M., Taliercio, V. L., Webber, L. B., Brandenberger, A. U., Rich, B. E., Beshay, A. P., Biber, J. E., Hess, R., Rhoads, J. L. W., & Secrest, A. M. (2022). The role of pain in the lives of patients with psoriasis: A qualitative study on an inadequately addressed symptom. *Journal of Psoriasis and Psoriatic Arthritis, 7*(1), 29–34. https://doi.org/10.1177/24755303211066928

Solmaz, N., Ilhan, N., & Bulut, H. M. (2021). The effect of illness perception on life quality in psoriasis patients. *Psychology, Health and Medicine, 26*(8), 955–967. https://doi.org/10.1080/13548506.2020.1847300

Stuewig, J., Tangney, J. P., Kendall, S., Folk, J. B., Meyer, C. R., & Dearing, R. L. (2015). Children's proneness to shame and guilt predict risky and illegal behaviors in young adulthood. *Child Psychiatry and Human Development, 46*(2), 217–227. https://doi.org/10.1007/s10578-014-0467-1

Svanström, C., Lonne-Rahm, S.-B., & Nordlind, K. (2019). Psoriasis and alcohol. *Psoriasis: Targets and Therapy, 9*, 75–79. https://doi.org/10.2147/PTT.S164104

Szepietowski, J. C., & Reich, A. (2016). Pruritus in psoriasis: An update. *European Journal of Pain (London, England), 20*(1), 41–46. https://doi.org/10.1002/ejp.768

Taliercio, V. L., Snyder, A. M., Webber, L. B., Langner, A. U., Rich, B. E., Beshay, A. P., Ose, D., Biber, J. E., Hess, R., Rhoads, J. L. W., & Secrest, A. M. (2021).

The disruptiveness of itchiness from psoriasis: A qualitative study of the impact of a single symptom on quality of life. *The Journal of Clinical and Aesthetic Dermatology, 14*(6), 42–48.

Tang, F.-Y., Xiong, Q., Gan, T., Yuan, L., Liao, Q., & Yu, Y.-F. (2022). The prevalence of alexithymia in psoriasis: A systematic review and meta-analysis. *Journal of Psychosomatic Research, 161*, 111017. https://doi.org/10.1016/j.jpsychores.2022.111017

Tangney, J. P., Wagner, P. E., Hill-Barlow, D., Marschall, D. E., & Gramzow, R. (1996). Relation of shame and guilt to constructive versus destructive responses to anger across the lifespan. *Journal of Personality and Social Psychology, 70*(4), 797–809. https://doi.org/10.1037/0022-3514.70.4.797

Thomsen, R. S., Nilsen, T. I. L., Haugeberg, G., Gulati, A. M., Kavanaugh, A., & Hoff, M. (2021). Adiposity and physical activity as risk factors for developing psoriatic arthritis: Longitudinal data from a population-based study in Norway. *Arthritis Care and Research, 73*(3), 432–441. https://doi.org/10.1002/acr.24121

Thomsen, S. F., Skov, L., Dodge, R., Hedegaard, M. S., & Kjellberg, J. (2019). Socioeconomic costs and health inequalities from psoriasis: A cohort study. *Dermatology, 235*(5), 372–379. https://doi.org/10.1159/000499924

Updike, J. (1985, February 9). At war with my skin. *New Yorker magazine.*

van der Vegte, K., Bremer-Ophorst, I., Bethlehem, S. A., Segers, L., Arets, B., & van Geelen, S. (2013). What is it like to be an adolescent with cystic fibrosis? Reversing the roles of patient and health-professional. *Journal of Cystic Fibrosis, 12*, S134. https://doi.org/10.1016/S1569-1993(13)60475-0

Wacewicz-Muczyńska, M., Socha, K., Soroczyńska, J., Niczyporuk, M., & Borawska, M. H. (2021). Cadmium, lead and mercury in the blood of psoriatic and vitiligo patients and their possible associations with dietary habits. *Science of the Total Environment, 757*, 143967. https://doi.org/10.1016/j.scitotenv.2020.143967

Warren, R. B., Kleyn, C. E., & Gulliver, W. P. (2011). Cumulative life course impairment in psoriasis: Patient perception of disease-related impairment throughout the life course. *British Journal of Dermatology, 164*, 1–14. https://doi.org/10.1111/j.1365-2133.2011.10280.x

Weiss, S. C., Kimball, A. B., Liewehr, D. J., Blauvelt, A., Turner, M. L., & Emanuel, E. J. (2002). Quantifying the harmful effect of psoriasis on health-related quality of life. *Journal of the American Academy of Dermatology, 47*(4), 512–518. https://doi.org/10.1067/mjd.2002.122755

Xiao, Y., Zhang, X., Luo, D., Kuang, Y., Zhu, W., Chen, X., & Shen, M. (2019). The efficacy of psychological interventions on psoriasis treatment: a systematic review and meta-analysis of randomized controlled trials. Psychology Research and Behavior Management, Volume 12, 97–106. https://doi.org/10.2147/PRBM.S195181

References

Yang, E., Beck, K., Sanchez, I., Koo, J., & Liao, W. (2018). The impact of genital psoriasis on quality of life: A systematic review. *Psoriasis: Targets and Therapy*, *8*, 41–47. https://doi.org/10.2147/PTT.S169389

Yang, S.-J., & Chi, C.-C. (2019). Effects of fish oil supplement on psoriasis: A meta-analysis of randomized controlled trials. *BMC Complementary and Alternative Medicine*, *19*(1), 354. https://doi.org/10.1186/s12906-019-2777-0

Zucchelli, F., Donnelly, O., Rush, E., White, P., Gwyther, H., Williamson, H., & VTCT Foundation Research Team at the Centre for Appearance Research. (2022). An acceptance and commitment therapy prototype mobile program for individuals with a visible difference: Mixed methods feasibility study. *JMIR Formative Research*, *6*(1), e33449. https://doi.org/10.2196/33449

Glossary of terms

Acceptance – the method of not resisting or struggling against negative thoughts or unpleasant feelings but instead accepting them.

Acceptance & Commitment Therapy (ACT) – a therapy which helps people put thoughts to one side and instead connect with the present and focus on what is important.

Alexithymia – a lack of awareness of one's emotional state with difficulties identifying and describing emotions (also known as emotional blindness).

Autonomic nervous system – a network of nerves controlling involuntary processes like heart rate, digestion and breathing, and constantly monitors the environment, taking account of what is going on in our bodies as well as our surroundings, to check whether things are safe.

Behavioural reactivation – purposely scheduling activity which brings feelings of pleasure and mastery.

Biologic treatment – a systemic treatment that reduces inflammation by targeting specific parts of the immune system rather than the entire immune system.

Cognitive Behavioural Therapy (CBT) – a therapy which helps people start to become more aware of their thought processes and then challenge unhelpful thinking.

Cognitive defusion – a strategy that allows you to take a step back from your thoughts and see them for what they are and not

Glossary of terms

what they say they are. This way you can observe them rather than be controlled by them.

Commitment – the method of taking action and making positive changes by considering values and what is important.

Drive system – feelings of motivation and striving that can be triggered by trying hard to accomplish a goal, like using treatments perfectly, sticking to a new diet or hiding skin.

Erythrodermic psoriasis – a rare form of the condition in which the whole body is affected by reddening of the skin and scaling.

Explain–Reassure–Distract – an effective method of managing comments and questions which can help reduce any feelings of distress triggered by unwanted attention.

Gate theory of pain – a theory which recognises the role of the brain in incorporating a range of information into the pain experience, such as past episodes of pain, levels of anxiety and attention.

Guttate psoriasis – psoriasis lesions which are small, drop-like and often extensive.

Illness beliefs – implicit beliefs about a health condition such as perceptions of symptoms and beliefs about what caused it, what consequences it will have and how long it will last.

Koebner phenomenon – psoriasis lesions occurring where there has been skin trauma or injury, such as a cut, an injection site or a burn.

Mindfulness – bringing your attention to the present moment, focusing on the here and now without judgement.

Negative bias – a bias towards negative thinking and paying more attention to negative experiences than positive experiences.

Orthorexia – a type of eating disorder where there is an obsessive focus on clean or healthy eating.

Phototherapy – a treatment using light waves. Either UVB, which is often delivered using a UVB cabinet in a hospital outpatient department or UVA, which is usually combined with a medication called psoralen and known as PUVA.

Glossary of terms

Plaque psoriasis – psoriasis lesions which are typically round in shape, a few centimetres in diameter, raised and covered in a silvery scale.

Polyvagal theory – a theory which describes how the autonomic nervous system monitors the environment and reacts to stress.

Psoriatic arthritis (PsA) – inflammation of the joints, tendons and ligaments.

Pustular psoriasis – psoriasis lesions which are characterised by pus-filled bumps or pustules.

Self-affirmation – using positive sentiments, like thinking about the things you value in yourself

Self-compassion – having kindness and compassion for yourself, in the same way you would show compassion for someone you love.

Soothe system – feelings of calm, relaxation and self-compassion that can be triggered by activities that foster feelings of safeness and contentment, like meditation, a relaxing walk or curling up with a good book and a hot drink.

Systemic treatment – drug therapies like tablets or injections that work throughout the whole body. Often an immunosuppressant medication designed to reduce the body's immune response and inflammation.

Thinking errors – also known as cognitive distortions, these are exaggerated ways of thinking that are not based on facts. Thinking errors can affect judgement, decision making and psychological well-being.

Threat system – feelings of arousal like panic, anger or disgust that can be triggered by self-criticism, shame, feeling exposed or judged.

About the author

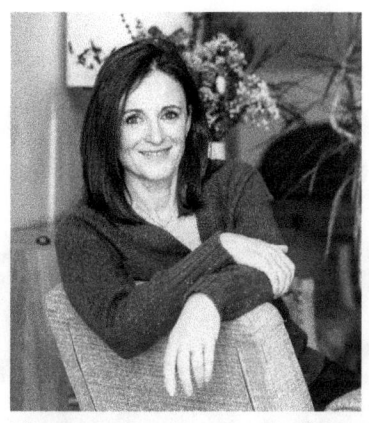

Photo credit: Gemma Griffiths.

Dr Catherine O'Leary is a consultant clinical psychologist who has worked for many years in medical settings in the NHS, including cleft lip and palate, renal and respiratory services. She has long wanted to use her expertise to help others with psoriasis but was never quite brave enough to tell the world about her condition. Thankfully, she has started to practise what she preaches, and in *Coping with Psoriasis*, Catherine shares her struggles with psoriasis and the psychological strategies that have helped her cope.

Catherine lives and works in South Wales and leads the psychology service at the All Wales Adult Cystic Fibrosis Service. She received her Ph.D. from the University of London and then went on to train as a clinical psychologist at the Institute of Psychiatry, King's College London. She is trained in several therapeutic approaches including Cognitive Behavioural Therapy, Family Therapy and Interpersonal Psychotherapy. She is passionate about supporting people and their families to live well with physical health conditions.